MW01118988

HELLO SLEEP, GOODNIGHT INSOMNIA: A 7 STEP DRUG FREE GUIDE UTILIZING CBT-I AND SLEEP HYGIENE TO SHARPEN FOCUS, ENHANCE PERFORMANCE, AND SUPPORT RESTFUL REJUVENATION AT ANY AGE

Bonuses: Cognitive Behavioral Therapy (CBT) Workbook, Sleep Supplement Guide, and 17 Short Boring Bedtime Stories Sure To Put Anyone Asleep

WILLIAM GRIST MD
YASMINE ELAMIR MD

© **Copyright 2024 - All rights reserved.**

The content contained within this book may not be reproduced, duplicated or transmitted without direct written permission from the author or the publisher.

Under no circumstances will any blame or legal responsibility be held against the publisher, or author, for any damages, reparation, or monetary loss due to the information contained within this book, either directly or indirectly.

Legal Notice:

This book is copyright protected. It is only for personal use. You cannot amend, distribute, sell, use, quote or paraphrase any part, or the content within this book, without the consent of the author or publisher.

Disclaimer Notice:

Please note the information contained within this document is for educational and entertainment purposes only. All effort has been executed to present accurate, up to date, reliable, complete information. No warranties of any kind are declared or implied. Readers acknowledge that the author is not engaged in the rendering of legal, financial, medical or professional advice. The content within this book has been derived from various sources. Please consult a licensed professional before attempting any techniques outlined in this book.

By reading this document, the reader agrees that under no circumstances is the author responsible for any losses, direct or indirect, that are incurred as a result of the use of the information contained within this document, including, but not limited to, errors, omissions, or inaccuracies.

CONTENTS

Dear Liam and Olivia:

You are our greatest motivation and living inspiration. Our commitment to healthy living is not only for our own well-being but also so that we can be present for every moment you grow, flourish, and chase your dreams. We love you like all little children love pennies.

Love always,
Mommy and Daddy.

INTRODUCTION

Your future depends on your dreams, so go to sleep. –

— MESUT BARAZANY

It's the dead of night, you've hit the pillow, and your body finally starts to wind down for some well-deserved rest. However, instead of your mind coasting into dreamland, it's speeding like a Formula 1 race car starting its final lap. Insomnia's got you in a chokehold. Sounds familiar? Well, you're not alone; in fact, you're part of a whopping 62% of adults who don't believe they're getting enough sleep (O'Reilly, 2019). Sleep deprivation has become a public health crisis and it's high time we confront this silent epidemic directly.

So, what motivated you to buy this book? What are you aiming to achieve? Maybe you were inspired by a particularly rough night when you felt like you'd tried everything and still couldn't find that elusive sleep. Perhaps you realized that your struggles with insomnia were affecting not just your health but your entire life. Whatever the catalyst, you're here now, and we get it. We understand where you are, what you're going through, and what you need.

Take this book as your guide to a better life through better sleep. By joining us on this journey, you're taking a shortcut to reclaiming your nights and revitalizing your days. You'll discover a comprehensive 7-step program that tackles insomnia from every angle, including cognitive behavioral therapy techniques, nutrition guidance, and stress management strategies. Imagine a life where you wake up refreshed, tackle your day with boundless energy, and nurture your well-being.

Now, let's dig deeper into the consequences of sleep deprivation. These are real health issues. Your memory struggles can lead to embarrassing situations, like forgetting your best friend's birthday or important meetings at work. Mood changes can strain your relationships, causing arguments and misunderstandings. Trouble with thinking and concentration can jeopardize your job performance, putting your career at risk. And let's not forget about your weakened immunity, which makes you more susceptible to catching every cold that passes by.

Enough doomsday talk; let's discuss the benefits of reading this book. By delving into these pages, you'll gain invaluable insights and shortcuts to transform your life. You're about to unlock the secrets to restorative sleep, enhanced productivity, and improved health. No more groggy mornings or sleepless nights; you're on the path to living your life to its fullest potential.

But why trust us? Good question. Let us introduce ourselves: We are Dr. Yasmine Elamir, a specialist in internal medicine and endocrinology, and Dr. William Grist, an expert in internal medicine and pulmonology. We're physicians dedicated to a healthy lifestyle in every facet of our lives. We've poured our medical expertise, personal experiences, and passion for well-being into this book. We have walked in your shoes, faced the same challenges, and emerged with evidence-based solutions that work.

Before we had the knowledge and strategies you'll find on these pages, we struggled with sleeping, too. We know how it feels to toss and turn night after night, yearning for the sweet embrace of sleep. We understand the frustration and physical effects that come with it. But we also know that transformation is possible when you have the right information and guidance.

So, let's make one thing crystal clear: This is not just another self-help book; it's a lifeline. It's the solution you've been searching for to conquer insomnia, improve your health, and revitalize your life.

So welcome to Hello Sleep, Goodnight Insomnia! Armed with science, humor, and a whole lot of heart, let's take the first steps on this expedition toward enhanced sleep and a more enriched life.

CHAPTER 1

THE IMPACT OF INSOMNIA
AND THE THREE-LETTER
SOLUTION

I find the nights long, for I sleep but little, and think much.

— CHARLES DICKENS

We once had a patient who struggled with insomnia. Her example was enlightening for us on a professional level, and that's why we want to share it with you. To protect this person's personal information, let's call her Sarah.

After a long struggle with insomnia, she discovered the 3-letter solution: CBT, which stands for cognitive behavioral therapy. A branch of this approach is cognitive behavioral therapy for insomnia (CBT-I) and sleep restriction. She decided to give it a shot, using an app from Stanford Medicine.

Before starting CBT-I, Sarah had been working on maintaining a consistent sleep-wake schedule. She stopped sleeping in on weekends and established a regular wake-up time.

The app she downloaded proved to be a valuable tool. It helped her challenge her old habits and establish new ones. No more hitting snooze for hours; she had moved beyond that phase. Her journey with CBT-I had begun, and she witnessed significant changes.

Implementing the technique of sleep restriction, Sarah started limiting her time in bed to match her actual sleep duration. This step substantially enhanced her sleep efficiency. Her bed was no longer associated with misery; it became a place of rest.

Over time, Sarah noticed progress. Her average sleep time began to approach six hours, a significant improvement. Although she understood that setbacks might occur, she appreciated the ability to fall asleep within minutes.

Sarah's journey wasn't a quick fix. It involved science-based strategies. Studies indicated that, when used in isolation, CBT-I had a success rate of 70–80% in mitigating insomnia symptoms. It was all part of a plan that aimed to change the long-standing connection between her bed and misery.

Reframing her self-talk and challenging unhelpful thoughts played a crucial role in her transformation. Positive self-talk helped her cope with sleep deprivation, reminding her that she had endured even more challenging days without sleep.

The Stanford app she embraced was instrumental. It allowed her to monitor her progress and reinforce CBT-I principles. Sarah had learned to recognize genuine signs of sleepiness, understanding when her body was truly ready for rest.

In the realm of sleep disorders, patience was key. Sarah aimed for the ultimate goal—seven hours of restful sleep. She knew it would take time and perseverance, but she was prepared for the journey ahead.

Sarah's story is not only about personal triumph; it also demonstrates the effectiveness of science-based strategies. Her journey shows that change is possible, even when it comes to something as personal as sleep. With the right tools and determination, restful nights are no longer a distant dream but a tangible reality.

This is the story of someone who, like you, suffered from insomnia and searched until she found a way to eradicate it. Your story may be similar. The first step will be to discover and analyze the biological and psychological foundations of this disorder. Thus, we will be prepared to cut this tree from the roots and ensure that it never again branches and disturbs our rest.

Let's explore the science behind sleeping and how to defeat insomnia forever.

THE HIDDEN CRISIS OF CHRONIC INSOMNIA

What Is Insomnia?

Insomnia is a sleep disorder characterized by difficulty falling asleep, staying asleep, or walking up early with difficulty getting back to sleep. It often leads to poor sleep quality, inadequate sleep duration, and daytime impairment in various aspects of functioning. Insomnia encompasses a range of symptoms, including difficulty falling asleep, frequent awakenings during the night, early morning awakenings, and a general sense of dissatisfaction with sleep (Roth, 2007).

Insomnia is undeniably a prevalent concern with a growing global impact, affecting a substantial percentage of the population. Credible research like that of Bhaskar et al. (2016) reveals the widespread nature of this issue, affecting an estimated 10–30% of people worldwide.

This nightly struggle doesn't stay confined to your bedroom; it spills over into your daily life with some serious consequences: First off, you're exhausted. The kind of tiredness where even the simplest tasks feel like climbing Mount Everest. It's as if a thick fog blankets your every move. Insomnia isn't just about tossing and turning in bed; it messes with your mind and body.

It's like being in a constant state of jet lag, where everything is out of sync. And it's not just physical; it messes with your emotions, too. Irritability and anxiety can turn minor annoyances into major dramas. Here's the kicker: These problems can both cause and result in insomnia. It's like a never-ending loop.

Now, let's dive into the various subtypes of insomnia to gain a comprehensive understanding of this complex condition. By understanding your unique subtype, you can also understand the unique treatment options at your disposal.

Acute Insomnia

Definition: Acute insomnia is a short-term sleep issue typically triggered by stress or specific life events, like exams or job interviews. It usually lasts less than three months and often resolves once the triggering event has passed.

Example: "The night before my job interview, I was tossing and turning, constantly glancing at the clock."

Solution: Implement relaxation techniques like progressive muscle relaxation or guided imagery to temporarily relieve stress and anxiety.

Chronic Insomnia

Definition: Chronic insomnia is a long-lasting sleep disturbance that occurs at least three nights a week and lasts three months or longer. It can severely impact your quality of life.

Example: "For the past six months, getting even just five hours of sleep feels like a win."

Solution: Medical consultation is advised. A healthcare provider may recommend a combination of medications and CBT-I.

Onset Insomnia

Definition: Onset insomnia manifests as difficulty in initially falling asleep. It involves trouble falling asleep despite feeling tired, leading to a prolonged period of wakefulness after bedtime, often due to racing thoughts or other reasons for a heightened state of arousal.

Example: "I get into bed exhausted, but my mind races, and sleep eludes me."

Solution: CBT-I includes behavioral changes like sleep restriction and stimulus control. You can start by creating a sleep-conducive environment that's cool, dark, and quiet to aid in falling asleep faster.

Maintenance Insomnia

Definition: Maintenance insomnia involves frequent awakenings after initially falling asleep. It's the inability to maintain sleep, characterized by repeated awakenings through the night and difficulty returning to sleep.

Example: "I wake up multiple times throughout the night, and it takes me an age to drift back to sleep."

Solution: Sleep restriction—a key component of CBT-I—is a behavioral intervention that limits the amount of time spent lying in bed to match the actual time spent sleeping. The goal here is to improve sleep efficiency and consolidate sleep.

Early Morning Awakening

Definition: Early morning awakening is when you wake up earlier than intended and can't go back to sleep. It involves awakening well before your desired wake-up time and being unable to return to sleep.

Example: "Even though my alarm is set for 7 a.m., I find myself awake and restless by 4:30 a.m."

Solution: Morning light therapy can help recalibrate your internal body clock, helping you wake up at a more reasonable hour. CBT-I can help retrain your body's internal clock. This includes strategies like stimulus control so the body only associates your bedroom with sleep and relaxation. Another method includes relaxation techniques to combat the heightened stress and anxiety that accompanies this type of insomnia.

The Detrimental Effects of Chronic Insomnia on Physical and Mental Health

The connection between sleep and mental health is firmly rooted in scientific evidence. When sleep quality is poor or insufficient, it can have a significant impact on our mental well-being. According to a study conducted by Morin et al. (2021), about 20% of people affected by a mental disorder in the United States suffered from insomnia before their diagnosis.

Chronic insomnia often leads to heightened irritability, making it easier to become frustrated and affecting our interactions with others. Mood swings become more frequent, rapidly shifting from happiness to sadness or frustration. Furthermore, poor sleep can contribute to increased anxiety and persistent worry, making it challenging to cope with daily stressors.

Over time, this persistent sleep deprivation can elevate the risk of developing depression, adding to the mental health burden (Fernandez-Mendoza & Vgontzas, 2013). Sleep plays a crucial role as a guardian of our emotional resilience behind the scenes. Inadequate sleep significantly impacts cognitive functions, making even simple tasks challenging and information retention difficult.

Beyond cognitive functions, sleep also regulates our emotions, influencing how we perceive and handle life's challenges. Scientific research, such as studies published in *Behavioral Sleep Medicine* (Taylor et al., 2003), highlights the heightened risk of mood disorders like depression and anxiety among those with chronic insomnia.

For individuals dealing with chronic insomnia, daily life can become a constant struggle with mood fluctuations, irritability, and exhaustion, making it difficult to manage even minor stressors. This clear link between insomnia and mental health underscores the urgency of addressing sleep-related issues for overall well-being, and it's firmly grounded in scientific research.

You might be thinking, So, *how do I achieve this?* Well, before jumping to practical strategies, it is necessary to know what the roots of this problem are to control them and achieve that long-awaited deep rest.

CAUSES AND TRIGGERS OF INSOMNIA

Stress is a common disruptor of sleep. It can lead to racing thoughts and anxiety, making it difficult to fall asleep (Suni, 2022). Irregular sleep patterns, such as constantly changing bedtime and wake-up times, can confuse your internal sleep clock, making it hard to establish a consistent sleep routine.

Your lifestyle choices, including your diet, exercise habits, and caffeine intake, can impact your sleep. For example, eating heavy or spicy meals close to bedtime, exercising vigorously late at night, or consuming caffeine can disrupt your sleep.

Mental health conditions like depression and anxiety can keep you awake due to emotional turmoil. Physical pain, whether from an injury or chronic condition, can cause discomfort that disrupts sleep.

Certain medications may interfere with sleep patterns, so it's important to find ones that don't. Neurological disorders, aging, and other sleep disorders can also disrupt sleep patterns. Pregnancy and menopause can introduce hormonal changes that lead to sleep disturbances, such as hot flashes and night sweats (Geng, 2021).

Now that we know exactly what insomnia is, what causes it, and how it impacts our health, it is time to continue our exploration and reveal the mystery of how to conquer insomnia once and for all. Let's go for it!

COGNITIVE BEHAVIORAL THERAPY: A SCIENCE-BACKED SOLUTION

At its core, CBT is a form of psychotherapy that emphasizes the powerful connection between thoughts, feelings, and behaviors. It recognizes that thoughts can influence emotions, which, in turn, can influence actions.

Here's how it works: CBT encourages you to become an active observer of your own thoughts, like a scientist conducting experiments within the laboratory of your mind. You'll learn to identify negative thought patterns and beliefs that may be contributing to your insomnia. Once identified, these patterns are gently challenged and replaced with more constructive and sleep-friendly thoughts.

CBT's effectiveness in addressing a wide range of mental health concerns led to the birth of a specialized branch: the aforementioned CBT-I. This tailored approach focuses specifically on the thoughts, behaviors, and habits that contribute to sleeplessness.

Now, you might wonder, does this approach really work? The answer is a resounding yes, backed by a robust body of scientific research. Numerous studies have shown that CBT-I is a highly effective treatment for insomnia. In fact, the American College of Physicians (2016) strongly recommends CBT-I as the first-line treatment for chronic insomnia. This is a testament to the therapy's proven track record of helping individuals regain control of their sleep patterns, with a success rate of 73% (Lamberg, 2016).

So, what are the key principles and techniques that make CBT-I so effective? Here's a glimpse into the tools you'll find in your CBT-I toolkit:

- **Sleep restriction:** Paradoxically, limiting your time in bed can improve sleep efficiency. By spending less time awake in bed, your body learns to associate the bed with sleep rather than wakefulness.
- **Stimulus control:** This technique helps break the association between bed and wakefulness. You'll learn to use the bed only for sleep and intimacy, not for activities like reading or watching TV.
- **Sleep hygiene:** Simple adjustments to your daily routines and sleep environment can significantly impact your sleep quality. We'll explore these tweaks in detail.
- **Cognitive restructuring:** This is the heart of CBT-I. You'll identify and challenge unhelpful thoughts about sleep, replacing them with a helpful narrative that serves you.
- **Relaxation techniques:** Stress and tension often contribute to insomnia. Learning relaxation exercises can help calm your mind and prepare your body for rest.

Don't panic! We don't expect you to know how to do all these things. We are actually introducing you to these as the foundations of CBT-I and will further expand on each one in the following chapters, which are directly used in our 7-step framework. We have even included a workbook in the bonus section so you can practice these skills and take them to the next level!

REAL-LIFE SUCCESS STORIES OF OVERCOMING INSOMNIA WITH CBT

Laura's journey:

Laura's story is a testament to the transformative power of CBT-I. For years, she battled chronic insomnia, watching her sleeplessness chip away at her well-being. Each night, she'd toss and turn, plagued by racing thoughts and restlessness. Mornings arrived, and she felt more like a zombie than a human being.

But Laura's turning point came when she stumbled upon CBT-I. With the guidance of a skilled therapist, she embarked on a journey of self-discovery. Laura learned to identify the anxious thoughts that had kept her awake for so long. As she challenged and reframed these thoughts, her sleep patterns gradually improved.

Through the practice of sleep restriction and stimulus control, Laura trained her body and mind to associate the bed with sleep once more. The nights of endless restlessness became a thing of the past. Laura's story serves as a reminder that even the most persistent insomnia can be conquered with the right tools and mindset.

Mark's battle with shift work insomnia:

Mark, a dedicated nurse, found himself wrestling with the unique challenge of shift work insomnia. His erratic work schedule wreaked havoc on his sleep patterns, leaving him exhausted and frustrated. It seemed impossible to find a rhythm that allowed for restful sleep.

CBT-I provided Mark with a sound solution. With the support of his therapist, he devised a personalized sleep plan tailored to his shift work schedule. Through sleep restriction and stimulus control, Mark gradually trained his body to adapt to his ever-changing hours. He learned relaxation techniques to ease the transition between work and sleep.

Mark's journey was not without its ups and downs, but his perseverance paid off. He regained control over his sleep, no longer held captive by the demands of his job. His story reminds us that even those facing unique sleep challenges can find solace and improve sleep through CBT-I.

Lucy's struggle with postpartum insomnia:

Lucy, a new mother, experienced the joys and challenges of parenthood, including postpartum insomnia. The demands of caring for her newborn left her sleep-deprived and frazzled. As exhaustion set in, she found herself unable to fall asleep even when her baby finally slept soundly.

CBT-I became Lucy's answer, offering her hope when sleeplessness threatened to consume her. She learned to recognize the anxious thoughts that plagued her mind during the night. With the guidance of her therapist, Lucy embraced cognitive restructuring, replacing those thoughts with soothing, sleep-promoting beliefs.

Through sleep hygiene adjustments and relaxation techniques, she gradually regained the precious hours of sleep she so desperately needed. Her story serves as a beacon of hope for sleep-deprived parents navigating the tumultuous waters of new parenthood.

We will explore the world of sleep hygiene, exploring the daily habits and rituals that can either hinder or enhance our quest for peaceful slumber. From the soothing power of a bedtime routine to the subtle influence of our sleep environment, every element plays a role in shaping our sleep quality.

CHAPTER 2

ESTABLISHING SLEEP
HYGIENE AND ROUTINES

A well-spent day brings happy sleep.

— LEONARDO DA VINCI

Imagine for a moment the feeling of waking up each morning, rejuvenated and ready to seize the day. Picture nights of uninterrupted, blissful sleep, where you effortlessly slip into dreamland, and rest wraps around you like a comforting cocoon. Now, consider this: The path to such restorative sleep begins with one fundamental concept—routines.

In this chapter, we embark on a journey to explore the critical role that routines play in the pursuit of quality sleep. We'll unravel the mysteries of sleep hygiene and discover practical strategies for crafting personalized sleep routines that will transform your nights, improve the quality of your sleep, and, consequently, your days.

INTRODUCTION TO SLEEP HYGIENE: A FOUNDATION FOR HEALTHY SLEEP

Much like you wouldn't skip brushing your teeth for a healthy smile, neglecting sleep hygiene can lead to a host of sleep-related problems. Poor sleep hygiene can disrupt your sleep patterns, leaving you fatigued, irritable, and less productive during the day.

Creating and adhering to a consistent routine is at the heart of good sleep hygiene. Just as you follow a daily schedule for meals, work, and leisure, establishing a regular sleep schedule is paramount. Going to bed and waking up at roughly the same times each day helps synchronize your body's internal clock, making it easier to fall asleep and wake up naturally.

Similarly, maintaining a clean and orderly living space and creating a conducive sleep environment is another essential aspect of sleep hygiene. A sleep-conducive environment includes factors such as dim lighting, an ideal thermostat temperature, and the absence of electronic devices in the bedroom. These elements work together to create a peaceful sanctuary where sleep can flourish.

Now, consider your caffeine intake as akin to selecting the right fuel for your body. Surely, you wouldn't put harmful substances into your vehicle's gas tank; consuming caffeine too close to bedtime can disrupt your sleep. To maintain good sleep hygiene, limit caffeine intake in the hours leading up to sleep, opting for decaffeinated alternatives if needed. It's best to stop caffeine intake at least six hours before sleep. However, for many, even this is not enough. We recommend going back two hours further each day if six hours is not enough or, even better, cutting caffeine altogether!

This chapter delves into the principles of sleep hygiene and offers practical strategies to establish personalized sleep routines that will pave the way for nights of restful slumber and days filled with vitality.

THE ESSENTIALS OF SLEEP SCHEDULES

Imagine your body has its internal clock, just like the ticking hands of a clock on the wall. This internal clock is called the circadian rhythm, and it regulates various bodily functions, including your heart rate, blood pressure, and more. Keeping a consistent sleep schedule is like winding that clock regularly, ensuring it runs smoothly.

Research shows that maintaining a consistent sleep schedule has numerous benefits (Moore, 2021). Firstly, it helps synchronize your body's internal clock, leading to better sleep quality and duration.

Here's why consistency matters: When you stick to a regular sleep schedule, your circadian rhythm remains stable.

Now, let's get into the details. Chronic sleep deprivation can throw a wrench into this well-oiled machine. When you don't get enough sleep, your body's secretion of human growth hormone (HGH) can be inhibited. HGH plays a crucial role in building lean muscle mass and burning fat. It's produced predominantly during the restful stage of sleep, known as slow-wave sleep.

So, when you're chronically sleep-deprived and missing out on that essential slow-wave sleep, your body produces less HGH. The consequence? Slower metabolism and potential weight gain. In essence, inconsistent sleep patterns can lead to unfavorable changes in your body's composition.

As you can see, consistency in sleep patterns offers a multitude of advantages. Let's explore some of them:

- **Optimal sleep quality:** When you go to bed and wake up at the same time each day, your body gets accustomed to this routine. It can prepare itself for sleep and wakefulness, resulting in more efficient and restorative sleep. Disruptions to your schedule can lead to fragmented or shallow sleep.
- **Synchronized hormonal release:** Your circadian rhythm influences the release of hormones such as melatonin and cortisol. Melatonin is responsible for promoting sleep, while cortisol is associated with wakefulness. Consistent sleep patterns ensure that these hormonal releases align with your sleep schedule, making it easier to fall asleep and wake up.
- **Improved sleep efficiency:** A regular sleep schedule improves sleep efficiency, which means you spend a higher percentage of your time in bed asleep. This results in better overall sleep quality and more restful nights.
- **Reduced jet lag:** Maintaining a consistent sleep schedule, especially when traveling across time zones, can help reduce the effects of jet lag. It allows your circadian rhythm to adjust gradually to the new time zone, minimizing sleep disturbances.
- **Enhanced alertness and performance:** When you consistently wake up at the same time, your body becomes accustomed to being alert and active during certain hours of the day. This can lead to improved cognitive performance, concentration, and daytime alertness.
- **Strengthened circadian rhythm:** Consistency reinforces your circadian rhythm, making it more resilient to external disruptions. It can help you adapt to changes in

daylight, shift work, or other lifestyle factors that may affect your sleep.

Now, let's delve into actionable strategies that seamlessly integrate a structured sleep schedule into the tapestry of your daily life, ensuring your nights are restful and your days are vibrant:

- **Set a consistent bedtime and wake-up time:** Choose a bedtime and wake-up time that you can realistically stick to, even on weekends. For example, if you decide to go to bed at 11 p.m. and wake up at 7 a.m., aim to follow this schedule consistently.
- **Prioritize sufficient sleep:** Assess your individual sleep needs and make sure you're getting at least 7 hours of sleep each night if you're an adult. Older adults over 60 may require 7–9 hours.
- **Establish a relaxing pre-sleep routine:** Create a soothing nightly routine that helps you unwind. This could involve activities like reading, taking a warm bath, practicing meditation, or gentle yoga.
- **Optimize your sleep environment:** Ensure your sleep space is conducive to rest. Turn off all electronics at least an hour before bedtime, keep your bedroom dark, and maintain a comfortable room temperature.
- **Incorporate physical activity:** Engage in regular physical activity to enhance both the quality and quantity of your sleep. For evening exercisers, avoid vigorous workouts within an hour of bedtime.
- **Gradual adjustments:** If you need to shift your sleep schedule, consider making incremental changes. Begin by moving your bedtime or wake-up time up or down by just 30 minutes every 3–4 days, making the transition smoother and more sustainable.

- **Comprehensive routine:** Maintaining a consistent timetable for your entire day, not just your sleep schedule, can greatly assist in sticking to your desired sleep pattern. This includes regular meal times and even other activities like exercise and intimate moments.
- **Track your habits:** If you encounter challenges in adhering to your sleep routine, keep a journal of your evening and morning activities. Analyzing this record can help you identify potential obstacles and make necessary adjustments to overcome them. For example, if you notice you had an afternoon diet coke that you normally don't have and had a poor night's sleep. Presto, you have figured out the potential source of your problem, which is likely the caffeine in the afternoon—yes, soda has caffeine.
- **Relaxing wind-down:** Establish a calming pre-sleep routine that doesn't involve electronic devices. To unwind before bedtime, engage in activities such as reading a book or practicing meditation. Additionally, reflect on your pre-sleep behaviors on nights when you have difficulty falling asleep—perhaps you are watching the Bachelor late at night or doom-scrolling on your Instagram feed.
- **Morning light exposure:** Exposure to natural daylight in the morning can facilitate waking up. Open your curtains or windows to allow the brightness of the morning sun into your room. Even better, go outside and take a walk in the morning. This is a reminder to your body and circadian rhythm to get up! Alternatively, consider using specialized glasses, like Luminette Glasses, designed to enhance your exposure to light and improve sleep quality.
- **Avoid sleep disturbances:** Be mindful of common sleep disruptors such as caffeine intake close to bedtime, late afternoon naps, and excessive exposure to blue light from electronic devices. Minimize these factors as much as

possible to protect the quality of your sleep. If you must use devices, consider wearing blue-light-blocking glasses to mitigate their impact.

- **Coordinate with your partner:** If you share a bed with a partner, communication is key. Discuss your respective bedtimes and wake-up times to ensure that you don't inadvertently disrupt each other's restful sleep. Consider noise cancellers for spouses who get up often at night to urinate or snore. If the last is the case, we recommend a sleep study for your partner.

Managing sleep when faced with schedule challenges, such as irregular work shifts, 24-hour shifts, or traveling across different time zones, requires specific strategies to ensure a good night's rest. Let's explore practical ways to overcome these hurdles:

When the **clocks spring forward** or **fall back,** it can disrupt your sleep schedule. To ease this transition:

- **Start shifting your schedule a week early:** Gradually adjust your bedtime and wake-up time by 15 minutes each day to align with the new time.
- **Modify caffeine intake:** Cut off caffeine an hour earlier than usual, and avoid alcohol, smoking, and intense exercise after dinner.
- **Stick to the new schedule:** Get up when the alarm rings, even if you're tired. Consistency helps your body adapt more quickly.
- **Embrace morning sunshine**: Sunlight in the morning can reset your internal clock and help you wake up more easily.

Traveling to **different time zones** can lead to jet lag, but there are ways to mitigate its effects:

- **Adjust to your destination:** Pretravel preparations should include adjusting your schedule an hour earlier or later, depending on your travel direction, if the trip is planned for a while. When heading westward, limit natural light exposure by using dark curtains and an eye mask and spending less time outdoors in the late afternoon and evening. This approach helps your body avoid thinking it's time to wind down. In contrast, when traveling eastward, aim to get natural light exposure early to wake you up and limit light exposure to help you fall asleep early. Avoid screen time to facilitate the adjustment.
- **Sync your eating schedule:** Align your meals with the local time of your destination to help reset your internal clock.
- **Prepare for jet lag symptoms:** Anticipate daytime sleepiness if it's daytime at your destination or nighttime insomnia if it's night. Be prepared for headaches, changes in appetite and digestion, and mood swings. To mitigate these symptoms, try to stay awake during the day and sleep at night while on a flight. Stay well-hydrated during the flight to counteract the common dehydration caused by low humidity. Avoid alcohol and caffeine in the air due to their dehydrating effects.
- **Be patient:** Your body clock shifts slowly, so it may take several days to fully adapt when crossing multiple time zones.

Those who work **irregular shifts** or night shifts can face unique sleep challenges. Here's how to navigate them:

- **Use bright light exposure:** To wake up during the night shift, expose yourself to blue light from devices or bright lights.
- **Consider small caffeine doses:** Consume small amounts of caffeine throughout your workday to help you stay alert.
- **Optimize your sleep environment:** Sleep in a dark, quiet room during the day and use light-blocking window coverings. Silence your phone.
- **Time your exercise and naps:** Exercise or nap during work breaks, but avoid doing so too close to bedtime.
- **Maintain a consistent routine:** Go to bed right after work, then follow your usual daily routine when you wake up. This includes adjusting your eating schedule to fit your day. Make sure to stop eating at least 2–3 hours before bed.
- **Adapt as needed:** Shift workers often need to be flexible to accommodate their schedules and maintain their well-being.

ROUTINES FOR SUCCESS

A bedtime routine offers a buffer zone between the hustle and bustle of daily life and the tranquility of sleep. It's a transition period during which you gradually detach from the day's stressors and demands. This unwinding process is vital, especially in today's fast-paced world.

Six hours before bedtime:

- Dinner: Have a light and balanced dinner. Avoid heavy, spicy, or fatty foods that can cause discomfort or indigestion.
- Hydration: Limit your fluid intake to avoid waking up for bathroom trips during the night.
- Caffeine and alcohol: Avoid caffeine and alcohol, as they can disrupt sleep patterns.

Four hours before bedtime:

- Screen time: Reduce exposure to screens, including smartphones, computers, and TVs. The blue light emitted from screens can interfere with melatonin production.
- Relaxation: Engage in calming activities like reading, gentle stretching, or deep breathing exercises to unwind.

Two hours before bedtime:

- Dim the lights: Create a relaxing atmosphere by dimming the lights in your home. This signals to your body that it's time to wind down.
- Warm bath or shower: Taking a warm bath or shower can help lower your body temperature, which aids in falling asleep.

One hour before bedtime:

- Screen-free zone: Continue to avoid screens. Consider switching to a traditional book or listening to soothing music.

Beyond the structured routine, let's ensure your bedroom is a sleep-conducive environment:

Bedroom environment:

- Make sure your bedroom is cool, dark, and quiet. Consider using blackout curtains if necessary.
- Invest in comfortable bedding, including a mattress and pillows that provide adequate support. You might even want to explore the calming effects of weighted blankets, which reduce anxiety and promote relaxation. For those who tend to get hot, options like cooling blankets, such as those from Evercool, can be considered.

Temperature:

- Maintain a comfortable room temperature, typically between 65–68°F (18–20°C).

These activities are not meant to be a checklist but a toolkit from which you can choose based on your preferences. You can mix and match them to create a personalized bedtime routine that suits you. The key is to prioritize relaxation, and over time, you'll find that your bedtime routine becomes a cherished part of your day.

The need for different amounts of sleep in individuals stems from a combination of factors, which encompass genetics, age, lifestyle, and overall health. Let's delve into these factors.

Genetics exerts a substantial influence on determining an individual's sleep requirements. Some individuals possess genetic predispositions that make them either more or less dependent on sleep (Sehgal & Mignot, 2011). This genetic diversity explains why certain people can thrive on just a few hours of rest while others necessitate a solid eight hours or even more.

Age is a pivotal factor in ascertaining the quantity of sleep an individual requires. As we progress through the various stages of life, our sleep demands evolve accordingly. Let's break it down by age group.

In the realm of children, infants and young children necessitate the most sleep. Newborns typically slumber for approximately 14–17 hours a day, gradually reducing this need to 9–11 hours as they transition into toddlerhood. School-age children typically require 9–11 hours of nightly rest to support their ongoing growth and development. While we don't cover this in this book, it is helpful to know if you are planning your sleep routine while juggling your children or grandchildren as well.

On average, adults need approximately 7–9 hours of sleep per night. However, it's vital to acknowledge individual variations. Some adults find themselves functioning optimally with just 6 hours of sleep, while others require a full 9 hours for peak performance.

For older people, sleep patterns tend to change as they age. They may experience more fragmented sleep, characterized by frequent awakenings throughout the night. While their sleep needs might decrease slightly, they still necessitate a restorative 7–8 hours of sleep (NIH, 2022).

Lifestyle factors can significantly impact an individual's sleep requirements. These encompass physical activity levels, dietary choices, and stress levels. Individuals engaged in vigorous physical activities may require more sleep to aid in recovery. At the same time, those with high-stress occupations may need additional rest to mitigate the impact of stress on sleep quality.

Furthermore, overall health plays a pivotal role in shaping sleep needs. Chronic illnesses, the use of certain medications, and the presence of sleep disorders can disrupt an individual's sleep patterns, potentially necessitating either more or less sleep to maintain overall well-being.

To optimize sleep health within each group, we need to go deeper into comprehensive guidelines and strategies.

For the young ones, consistency is paramount. They thrive on routines, so establishing a consistent bedtime that aligns with the recommended sleep duration for their age is essential. The National Sleep Foundation suggests varying sleep durations based on age: preschoolers (3–5 years) require 10–13 hours, school-age children (6–13 years) should aim for 9–11 hours, and teenagers (14–17 years) benefit from 8–10 hours of nightly sleep (Hirshkowitz et al., 2015).

Another critical facet of sleep hygiene for children is limiting screen time before bedtime. The blue light emitted from electronic devices can interfere with their ability to fall asleep as it suppresses melatonin production (Lee et al., 2018). It's prudent to establish a screen curfew, allowing ample time for the circadian rhythm to adjust.

Moreover, cultivating a relaxing bedtime routine is beneficial. Engaging in calming activities like reading a bedtime story, practicing relaxation exercises, or taking a warm bath can help children wind down and transition into a peaceful slumber.

Additionally, attention to the sleep environment is vital. Ensuring a comfortable sleep space with a cozy mattress and maintaining an appropriate room temperature promotes restful sleep.

For adults, sleep hygiene pivots on several key principles. Prioritizing sleep duration within the range of 7–9 hours, based on individual needs and preferences, is crucial. It's important to acknowledge that sleep requirements vary among individuals, so experimentation may be necessary to determine the ideal amount of sleep (American Academy of Sleep Medicine, 2015).

Consistency in the sleep schedule is another cornerstone. Maintaining a regular sleep-wake pattern, even on weekends, helps regulate the circadian rhythm, reinforcing the body's internal clock (Markwald et al., 2018).

Furthermore, managing stimulants is pivotal. Avoiding caffeine and heavy meals close to bedtime, along with reducing alcohol consumption, is recommended to prevent sleep disturbances.

Integrating relaxation techniques, such as meditation or deep breathing exercises, into the bedtime routine aids in stress management, fostering a tranquil pre-sleep state.

Lastly, the sleep environment must be conducive to restorative sleep. A bedroom should ideally be dark, quiet, and set at a comfortable temperature to promote uninterrupted slumber.

Older adults face unique challenges related to sleep hygiene. It's important to recognize that sleep patterns may naturally change with age, often resulting in fragmented nighttime sleep. To compensate for this, short naps during the day can be beneficial as long as they don't interfere with nighttime sleep (National Institute on Aging, 2017).

Additionally, limiting fluid intake before bedtime helps minimize nighttime awakenings to use the restroom, a common issue among older adults.

Engaging in regular physical activity is essential for older adults, but they should avoid vigorous exercise close to bedtime to prevent overstimulation.

Reviewing medications with a healthcare provider is also advised, as some medications may interfere with sleep. Adjusting the timing of medications, if feasible, can mitigate these disruptions.

Lastly, managing stress becomes even more critical for older adults, who may face unique stressors related to aging. Practicing stress management techniques, such as mindfulness meditation or engaging in fulfilling hobbies, can be beneficial.

THE ROLE OF LIGHT EXPOSURE

Light is a potent regulator of our internal biological clock or circadian rhythm. The suprachiasmatic nucleus (SCN) in the brain, often referred to as the body's "master clock," is highly sensitive to light. It receives signals from the retina in our eyes, particularly the blue wavelengths of light, which are most effective at stimulating the SCN. When exposed to natural sunlight during the day, the SCN sends signals to suppress the production of melatonin, a hormone that induces sleepiness. This results in increased alertness and wakefulness (Blume et al., 2019).

Conversely, as the evening approaches and light exposure diminishes, the SCN signals the pineal gland to release melatonin, promoting drowsiness and facilitating the transition into sleep. Therefore, exposure to bright natural light during the day is essential for maintaining a healthy circadian rhythm, which, in turn, promotes better sleep at night.

Incorporating these findings into daily routines involves exposing oneself to natural sunlight, especially in the morning. Spending time outdoors for at least 30 minutes in the morning can help synchronize your internal clock and improve sleep quality. Additionally, minimizing exposure to artificial light sources, especially blue light from screens, in the evening hours can further support a smooth transition to sleep. Utilizing blue light filters on electronic devices or wearing blue-light-blocking glasses can be effective strategies.

Regular physical activity is another influential factor in sleep regulation. Exercise has been shown to enhance the quality and duration of sleep. Engaging in moderate aerobic activities, such as walking or jogging, increases the amount of deep sleep, which is essential for physical and mental restoration (Kline et al., 2014).

One of the mechanisms through which exercise promotes better sleep is its ability to reduce anxiety and stress. Physical activity triggers the release of endorphins, which act as natural mood lifters. This can alleviate symptoms of anxiety and depression, both of which are often associated with sleep disturbances.

LIGHT EXPOSURE

Let's break this into smaller pieces.

As we addressed before, natural sunlight plays a pivotal role in synchronizing our circadian rhythms.

Conversely, artificial light, especially blue light emitted by devices like cell phones, tablets, and laptops, can have a disruptive effect on our sleep. Blue light has a short wavelength and significantly impacts melatonin and circadian rhythms. Excessive evening use of such devices can lead to sleep problems (Tosini et al., 2016).

Even low levels of indoor light can affect our circadian rhythms. Research indicates that closing your eyes isn't sufficient to block out light, and the effects on circadian rhythm can persist.

The consequences of excessive artificial light exposure during sleep extend beyond sleep quality. They include eye strain, which can result in discomfort and difficulty focusing, weight gain due to disrupted circadian regulation of metabolism, and even potential associations with cancer risk (Tosini et al., 2016).

To adjust your bedroom environment for better sleep, consider these steps:

- **Motion-activated lights:** For trips to the bathroom at night, use motion-activated lights to provide necessary illumination without flooding your bedroom with light.
- **Consider an eye mask:** If a partner insists on having a light on or the TV on, wearing a close-fitting eye mask can help you sleep in darkness.
- **Change TV settings:** If you have a TV in the bedroom, consider removing it or using a sleep timer to turn it off automatically after a set time.
- **Limit screen time:** Minimize electronic device use by two to three hours before bedtime. Some devices offer a "night mode" to reduce blue light emission, or you can use apps that filter blue light.

COMMON SLEEP HYGIENE MISCONCEPTIONS

Sleep is a mysterious realm, and it's no wonder that misconceptions and myths have sprouted around it. In this section, we'll debunk some of the most common sleep myths and provide evidence-based corrections to help you improve your sleep hygiene.

You need a minimum of eight hours of sleep each night:

This myth suggests everyone should strive for a solid eight hours of sleep every night. While sleep recommendations indeed fall within the range of 7–9 hours for most adults, the key isn't the exact number of hours but rather the number of complete sleep cycles you experience. A full sleep cycle typically takes around 90 minutes to complete, encompassing four stages: being awake, light sleep, deep sleep, and rapid eye movement (REM) sleep (Patel & Araujo, 2018). Still, generally, most people need 4–5 hours to get there. Four cycles would amount to about 6 hours of sleep, and 5 cycles equates to about 7.5 hours of sleep, which falls into the recommended 7–9 hours, according to the American Academy of Sleep Medicine and the Sleep Research Society. Six cycles result in 9 hours of sleep.

Instead of obsessing over hitting a specific number of hours, focus on allowing yourself enough time to go through multiple sleep cycles. While this can vary from person to person, what's important is waking up feeling refreshed and maintaining that energy throughout the day.

It's normal to sleep less as we age:

While it's true that sleep patterns can change as we age, the misconception here is that older adults necessarily need less sleep. Aging brings alterations in hormonal levels and circadian rhythms, which can result in more awakenings during the night. However, this doesn't necessarily mean that older adults need less sleep.

Quality of sleep remains vital, and older adults should aim for 7–8 hours of restorative sleep. It's essential to adapt sleep habits to accommodate changes in sleep patterns and prioritize sleep hygiene as you age.

You can make up for lost sleep on weekends:

Many people believe they can compensate for weekday sleep deficits by sleeping in on weekends. While occasional deviations from your sleep schedule won't harm you, regularly shifting your sleep patterns can disrupt your circadian rhythm, making it harder to fall asleep and wake up at the right times.

Alcohol before bed improves rest:

This myth suggests that a nightcap can help you fall asleep faster. While alcohol might initially make you drowsy, it leads to disrupted sleep patterns later in the night. It's crucial to time alcohol consumption correctly, allowing a buffer of at least four hours between drinking and bedtime to avoid sleep disruptions.

More sleep is always better:

While adequate sleep is crucial, more isn't always better. For most adults, the ideal amount of sleep typically falls within the range of 6–9 hours. Sleeping excessively, especially beyond nine hours regularly, may indicate underlying health concerns.

Your goal should be to find your sweet spot for sleep duration, where you wake up feeling well-rested and maintain consistent sleep patterns.

Sleep problems are not very common:

Sleep problems are more widespread than you might think. Insomnia alone affects about 30% of the adult American population, with 10% experiencing severe impacts on their daily lives.

Many other sleep disorders and health conditions can also disrupt sleep quality (Colten & Altevogt, 2006).

If you're struggling with sleep issues, you're not alone. If necessary, ask your physician for a sleep study. Effective solutions are available to improve sleep quality and overall well-being.

Sleeping with a light on is harmless:

A common misconception is that sleeping with a light on has no adverse effects. In reality, even small amounts of light can disrupt sleep cycles, leading to nighttime awakenings and reduced sleep quality. To optimize sleep, create a dark, quiet, and cool sleep environment.

It doesn't matter what time of day you sleep:

While modern lifestyles sometimes lead to irregular sleep schedules, aligning your sleep with natural circadian rhythms is beneficial. Your body has an internal clock that influences when you feel alert and when you feel sleepy. Sleeping at night, when it's dark, promotes better sleep quality and helps maintain a consistent sleep schedule.

Now that we've dispelled common sleep myths and clarified the foundations of good sleep hygiene, it's time to delve deeper into the interconnected web of factors that influence our slumber. Just as a well-structured bedtime routine can set the stage for quality sleep, so too can our diet and lifestyle choices play pivotal roles in the quality of our rest.

In the following chapters, we'll explore how the food we eat, the activities we engage in, and the choices we make during our waking hours impact the quantity and quality of our sleep. Prepare to uncover the surprising ways in which your lifestyle can either enhance or hinder your sleep and discover practical strategies to optimize your daily routine for better nights and brighter mornings. You will be learning valuable insights into how your daily choices and your nightly rest are deeply entwined. By making the right choices expect profound improvement in your sleep!

CHAPTER 3

LIFESTYLE ADJUSTMENTS
FOR QUALITY SLEEP

It is a common experience that a problem difficult at night is resolved in the morning after the committee of sleep has worked on it.

— JOHN STEINBECK

These words beautifully encapsulate the mysterious yet transformative power of sleep. As we venture into this chapter, we find ourselves at the intersection of two vital aspects of our lives: our daily choices and the profound influence they wield over the quality of our slumber.

As Steinbeck suggests, sleep often acts as a silent committee, working tirelessly during the night to untangle the threads of our daily challenges and weave them into solutions. But what if we could empower this committee and provide it with the tools it needs to operate more effectively? That's precisely what this chapter aims to explore.

We'll journey into the world of lifestyle adjustments, uncovering the ways our diet and daily activities can either harmonize with the committee of sleep or disrupt its delicate deliberations. Through evidence-based insights and practical guidance, we'll navigate the terrain of food, exercise, and daily routines, illuminating the pathways to improved sleep and overall well-being.

THE INTRICATE DANCE OF DIET AND SLEEP

Next, we will unravel the intricate dance of diet and sleep, exploring how the foods we consume affect the quality of our slumber.

At its core, nutrition is the art and science of providing the body with the nourishment required to function optimally. It's the fuel that powers every cell, every thought, and every step of our daily journey. However, much like a personalized playlist, each of us has unique nutritional needs dictated by a medley of factors.

Age, gender, activity level, and even genetic predispositions all contribute to the symphony of our nutritional requirements. Just as a growing child needs different nutrients compared to an active young adult or a seasoned elder, our dietary needs are as diverse as the notes in a musical composition.

Now, imagine that sleep is the serene pause between movements in this grand symphony of life. It's during these moments of rest that our bodies repair, recharge, and recalibrate. But what happens when the conductor, nutrition, wields its baton with dissonance rather than harmony?

In the world of slumber, diet is the silent composer of your sleep quality. Just as a misplaced note can disrupt a melodious tune, poor dietary choices can disrupt your sleep patterns and, in turn, your overall well-being. Conversely, a well-composed diet can be the lullaby that serenades you into a peaceful night's rest.

Now, imagine a different scenario—one where your dietary choices are aligned with the sweet serenade of nutritious sleep.

In the following sections, we will delve deeper into the specific nutrients and dietary practices that can either elevate or disrupt the quality of your sleep. Like an orchestra perfecting its performance, we'll explore how you can fine-tune your diet to create a harmonious symphony of sleep, ensuring that the committee of sleep has the best resources to resolve the night's challenges by morning's light.

NUTRIENTS THAT NURTURE SLEEP

As we continue our exploration of the intricate relationship between diet and sleep, it's time to focus our attention on the specific nutrients that play pivotal roles in promoting a restful night's slumber.

Let's begin with tryptophan, often regarded as the maestro of sleep-promoting nutrients. This compound conducts an orchestra of serotonin and melatonin in the brain. Serotonin, known for its mood-enhancing properties, is the precursor to melatonin, the hormone that regulates our sleep-wake cycles (Binks et al., 2020).

Imagine tryptophan as the conductor of a symphony, guiding serotonin to create the peaceful overture of relaxation. It's found in various foods, and by including them in your diet, you can encourage the production of serotonin, ultimately leading to improved sleep.

You can find it in the following foods:

- turkey
- chicken
- cheese
- nuts (especially almonds)
- seeds (such as pumpkin and sunflower seeds)
- tofu
- salmon

Now, consider magnesium as the conductor of muscle relaxation. This essential mineral has a calming effect on both the nervous system and the muscles. It acts as a natural sedative, preparing your body for a peaceful night's sleep.

Think of magnesium as the gentle strings of a cello, soothing tense muscles and helping to reduce nighttime restlessness. Incorporating magnesium-rich foods into your diet can ease muscle tension and promote relaxation, aiding your quest for better sleep.

Some foods rich in magnesium are:

- leafy greens (like spinach and kale)
- nuts (such as almonds and cashews)
- seeds (like pumpkin seeds)
- whole grains (including brown rice and oats)
- dark chocolate (in moderation, of course)

Finally, picture melatonin as the conductor of the sleep-wake orchestra. This hormone, produced naturally by your body's pineal gland, helps regulate your circadian rhythm. It signals to your body that it's time to sleep and wake.

Melatonin's role can be likened to that of a conductor's baton, guiding your body through the phases of sleep. While it's produced naturally, certain foods can enhance its production and encourage a smoother transition into sleep.

Foods that support melatonin production:

- cherries
- grapes
- tomatoes
- olive oil
- walnuts

While we've explored the foods that can serenade you into sleep, it's equally important to identify those that can disrupt your journey to dreamland. Just as a jarring, dissonant note can disrupt a musical performance, certain dietary choices can sabotage your sleep quality.

Here are some foods and beverages to avoid before bedtime and the reasons behind their disruptive influence:

- **Spicy and fatty foods:** These can cause acid reflux and indigestion, making it difficult to sleep comfortably. Try not to consume spicy or fatty meals within three hours of bedtime.
- **High-sugar foods:** Sugary snacks and desserts can lead to blood sugar spikes and crashes, disrupting sleep. Avoid excessive sugar intake before bedtime.

By paying attention to the nutrients that nurture sleep and making thoughtful dietary choices, you can compose a diet that harmonizes with your body's natural rhythms, allowing the committee of sleep to work its magic throughout the night, just as John Steinbeck eloquently described.

Fasting and Rest

Fasting, for various reasons, has been a part of human culture and tradition for centuries. For some, it's a religious practice deeply intertwined with faith and spirituality. For others, it's a dietary regimen, often in the form of intermittent fasting, to achieve specific health goals. While fasting can have benefits for both the body and mind, it's essential to consider its potential impact on sleep.

For those who fast for religious reasons, maintaining the balance between spiritual devotion and physical well-being is crucial. Fasting during specific periods, like Ramadan for Muslims or Yom Kippur for Jews, can be a deeply meaningful experience. However, it's essential to pay attention to how fasting might affect your sleep patterns. During these fasts, the eating and drinking schedule changes significantly, often involving pre-dawn meals (Suhoor) and evening-breaking fast meals (Iftar). Ensuring that these meals provide proper nutrition, including adequate protein and complex carbohydrates, can help stabilize blood sugar levels and, in turn, support better sleep.

The timing of your last meal of the day becomes especially important when fasting. For those following intermittent fasting, where eating is restricted to a specific window of hours, it's advisable to have your last meal well before bedtime. Ideally, this meal should be consumed at least a few hours before you plan to sleep, as a full stomach can make falling asleep uncomfortable. Aiming for a cutoff time around 6 p.m. or earlier is a good practice, as it gives your body enough time to digest and process the food before bedtime.

Starting a new fasting routine or adjusting an existing one can have varying effects on sleep. When the body is accustomed to a particular eating schedule, changes in that routine can initially disrupt sleep patterns. This is particularly true for those adopting intermittent fasting or time-restricted eating. As your body adapts to the new schedule, you may experience temporary disturbances in sleep. It's essential to recognize that these disturbances are often a part of the adjustment process. As your body acclimates to the fasting routine, sleep patterns typically normalize.

Hydration is another critical factor to consider when fasting. Dehydration can lead to discomfort and restlessness during sleep. For those fasting, especially during long periods, it's essential to ensure proper hydration during non-fasting hours. This not only contributes to better sleep quality but also supports overall health.

THE TRUTH ABOUT CAFFEINE AND ALCOHOL

In exploring the effects of caffeine and alcohol on sleep from a biological and neurological perspective, we find a fascinating interplay between these substances and our sleep patterns. Caffeine, a widely consumed stimulant, can boost vigilance, but its prolonged presence in the system can disrupt sleep.

Caffeine operates as a double-edged sword, especially when it comes to sleep. At its core, caffeine works by blocking adenosine, a neurotransmitter in the brain responsible for promoting sleep and relaxation. Over the course of the day, adenosine levels naturally increase, contributing to the growing sense of tiredness you feel by evening. Caffeine's molecular structure allows it to fit into the same receptors in the brain as adenosine, effectively blocking adenosine's sleep-inducing action. This leads to increased alertness and wakefulness, as caffeine temporarily overrides the brain's natural signals for sleep (Lazarus et al., 2011).

Moreover, caffeine stimulates the release of neurotransmitters like dopamine and norepinephrine. (Alasmari, 2020) These chemicals are associated with improved mood and heightened cognitive function, further enhancing your sense of alertness and focus.

So, when you enjoy a cup of coffee to combat jet lag, for instance, you're essentially hijacking your brain's natural sleep-regulating mechanisms. This is why caffeine can be a valuable tool for shift workers, travelers adjusting to different time zones, or individuals facing occasional sleep disruption.

Nonetheless, while caffeine can help you stay awake when necessary, it's essential to understand its limitations and potential drawbacks.

Caffeine's half-life—the time it takes for half of it to be eliminated from your body—varies from person to person but is typically around 3–7 hours. This means that even several hours after your last cup of coffee, a significant amount of caffeine may still be active in your system. As a result, consuming caffeine in the afternoon or evening can interfere with your ability to fall asleep and stay asleep during the night (Lazarus et al., 2011).

Chronic or excessive caffeine intake can lead to sleep disturbances. It may reduce the overall amount of deep sleep, also known as slow-wave sleep, which is essential for physical restoration and memory consolidation. Rapid eye movement (REM) sleep, a phase associated with dreaming and cognitive processing, can also be affected, leading to fragmented and less restful sleep.

Alcohol, although widely consumed and often associated with relaxation, is a substance that can have detrimental effects on the brain and sleep (Brower, 2001).

Recent studies have brought to light the sobering reality that even moderate alcohol consumption can negatively affect brain health. One such study found that consuming just over half a standard drink per day—equivalent to roughly four grams of alcohol—was associated with a reduction in brain volume over time.

Daviet and his colleagues in 2022, It's like willingly signing up for a double whammy of brain aging and compromised sleep quality, a decision that simply doesn't make sense. The trade-off doesn't add up—it's a no-brainer.

Physiologically, alcohol disrupts various aspects of sleep. Let's explore them next.

While alcohol can initially make you feel drowsy and may seem like a shortcut to falling asleep, this is misleading. The sedative effects of alcohol act on the central nervous system, slowing down brain activity. However, this leads to lower-quality sleep as the night progresses. A study by Pietilä et al. (2018) found that these sedative effects result in shallower sleep patterns and frequent awakenings.

It also significantly adversely affects the REM (rapid eye movement) phase of sleep, which is critical for memory consolidation and cognitive function. Reduced REM sleep can lead to fewer dream experiences and impaired cognitive processes.

Persistent alcohol consumption can give rise to chronic sleep issues, particularly insomnia symptoms. According to research by Park et al. (2015), individuals may develop tolerance to alcohol's sedative effects, requiring more alcohol to initiate sleep. This pattern exacerbates existing sleep problems and leads to a cycle of dependency on alcohol for sleep.

Alcohol has a direct impact on the central nervous system. It acts as a sedative, slowing brain activity and altering neurotransmitter function. This may initially create a sense of relaxation, but it ultimately leads to a lower quality of sleep. As the body metabolizes alcohol throughout the night, it can cause frequent awakenings and an overall shallower sleep pattern (Pietilä et al., 2018).

Long-term alcohol misuse has also been linked to chronic sleep problems. Those with alcohol use disorders often report insomnia symptoms. Tolerance to alcohol can develop rapidly, leading individuals to consume more alcohol to initiate sleep. This ongoing pattern can exacerbate sleep issues and contribute to a cycle of dependency on alcohol to achieve sleep (Park et al., 2015).

Another significant concern is the relationship between alcohol and sleep apnea, a disorder characterized by abnormal breathing and temporary loss of breath during sleep. Alcohol relaxes the muscles in the throat, which can exacerbate obstructive sleep apnea symptoms. Studies have shown that alcohol increases the risk of sleep apnea by 25%, particularly if consumed before bedtime (Park et al., 2015).

While it may seem to offer short-term relief from stress or sleeplessness, its long-term impact on sleep quality and brain health cannot be ignored.

To learn more about alcohol's effects on health, including its impact on sleep and brain function, it's valuable to consult reputable resources and studies. Organizations like the National Institute on Alcohol Abuse and Alcoholism (NIAAA) provide comprehensive information on the subject. Understanding the science behind alcohol's influence on sleep can empower individuals to make informed choices regarding their consumption, ultimately promoting better sleep and overall well-being.

And What About Smoking?

The impact of smoking on sleep is a topic that warrants close attention, as it affects not only sleep quality but overall health. Smoking is a known contributor to a plethora of health issues, and its consequences extend into the realm of sleep.

One of the ways smoking affects sleep is by reducing the oxygen-carrying capacity of the blood, leading to a condition known as erythrocytosis. Erythrocytosis is characterized by an excess of red blood cells, which thickens the blood and raises the risk of clot formation and smoke. Some of their consequences are (McMullin, 2012):

- The heightened viscosity of the blood places added stress on the heart, potentially resulting in palpitations and nighttime breathlessness, thereby disturbing the quality of sleep.
- Individuals with erythrocytosis face an elevated risk of developing sleep apnea, which, in turn, can give rise to symptoms like snoring, choking, and recurrent nighttime awakenings.
- While an increase in blood cell count boosts oxygen saturation, the effective oxygenation of body tissues may decrease, potentially compromising the quality of sleep.
- This condition also contributes to heightened fatigue and weakness, making it more challenging to initiate or sustain sleep due to physical discomfort and restlessness.

Smoking's harmful effects on the respiratory system are well-documented. Chronic obstructive pulmonary disease (COPD) and asthma are two respiratory conditions that often worsen due to smoking. COPD, a progressive lung disease that includes chronic bronchitis and emphysema, can result in breathlessness and hinder the ability to maintain restful sleep.

Asthma, characterized by airway inflammation and bronchocon-striction, may lead to nighttime symptoms like coughing and wheezing, further disrupting sleep patterns. To manage these conditions effectively, individuals may rely on treatments that include inhaled steroids and bronchodilators, such as albuterol, to alleviate symptoms and improve lung function.

While these treatments are essential for managing COPD and asthma symptoms, they can introduce additional challenges for individuals trying to maintain healthy sleep patterns. Steroids, often a cornerstone of treatment, have been associated with insulin resistance and weight gain. This is particularly significant, as insulin resistance and obesity are known contributors to sleep apnea, a sleep disorder characterized by repetitive interruptions in breathing during sleep.

Albuterol, a common bronchodilator used to relieve asthma symp-toms, is known to have stimulating properties. This can affect sleep patterns, potentially leading to difficulties falling or staying asleep. The combination of these factors underscores the complex relationship between smoking, respiratory conditions, and sleep disturbances (CDC, 2020).

Studies have found a direct association between smoking and poor sleep quality, including disruptions in sleep architecture and decreased REM sleep duration, compromising crucial cognitive function and memory consolidation (Li et al., 2020).

Understanding the detrimental effects of smoking on sleep and overall health provides an opportunity for change. Smoking is not just a habit but a complex addiction with multifaceted conse-quences. It's a challenge, but it can be overcome. If you or someone you know is struggling with smoking, consider seeking assistance from smoking cessation programs, healthcare professionals, or support groups.

Quitting smoking is a compassionate act of self-care, a journey toward better sleep, improved health, and an enhanced quality of life. Remember, the path to change may not be easy, but it is undoubtedly worth the effort. Your sleep and well-being are precious; nurturing them is a decision that can transform your life.

EXERCISE: YOUR WAY TO BETTER SLEEP

We've explored how the quality of sleep can affect our physical well-being, but it's equally important to understand how exercise can reciprocate, nurturing our slumber in return.

Regular physical activity yields numerous benefits, encompassing a lower risk of diseases like cancer and diabetes, improved physical function, and an enhanced quality of life. Exercise also benefits specific groups; for instance, pregnant individuals who maintain regular physical activity are less likely to experience excessive weight gain or postpartum depression, while older adults who engage in exercise reduce their risk of fall-related injuries.

One significant benefit of exercise is its positive impact on sleep. Moderate to vigorous physical activity can substantially enhance sleep quality for adults by reducing sleep onset time—the time it takes to fall asleep—and decreasing the duration of nighttime wakefulness. Additionally, physical activity can mitigate daytime sleepiness and, in some cases, decrease the reliance on sleep medications.

Exercise can also indirectly enhance sleep by decreasing the risk of excessive weight gain. Excessive weight gain can contribute to obstructive sleep apnea (OSA), and roughly 60% of moderate to severe OSA cases have been linked to obesity, although this relationship is multifaceted (McMullin, 2012).

Studies conducted on diverse demographic groups have examined the effects of exercise on sleep quality. One study focused on college students during exam periods and found that exercise and physical activity can reduce test-related stress (Zhang et al., 2022). Another study highlighted the dynamic relationship between sleep and exercise for older adults in the community (Seol et al., 2021). A third study demonstrated that regular aerobic exercise can alleviate symptoms in individuals with OSA, irrespective of weight loss (Peng et al., 2022).

In contrast, jobs involving manual labor may not provide the same sleep benefits as exercise. Such laborious jobs often result in musculoskeletal discomfort that can adversely affect sleep. Additionally, long hours of manual labor can increase the risk of stress and fatigue among employees.

Aerobic exercises, such as brisk walking, jogging, swimming, or cycling, have been substantiated by research as potent tools for enhancing sleep quality. Engaging in these activities elevates your heart rate and breathing, facilitating the distribution of oxygen throughout your body. This increased circulation aids in the recovery and rejuvenation of muscles, laying the foundation for a restful night's sleep (National Heart, Lung, and Blood Institute, 2022). A highly accessible form of aerobic exercise for individuals of various fitness levels is brisk walking. Whether you are a novice or a seasoned exerciser, walking can be tailored to your fitness level.

Cardiovascular workouts, a subset of aerobic exercises, have been shown to boost both heart health and sleep quality. Activities like running, dancing, or engaging in jump rope workouts not only enhance cardiovascular fitness but also stimulate the release of endorphins, the body's natural mood enhancers, promoting relaxation and improved sleep. For those new to cardiovascular workouts, low-impact options like dancing or water aerobics are gentle on the joints while still delivering cardiovascular benefits. Gradually intensify your workouts as you build endurance, aiming for a minimum of 150 minutes of moderate-intensity cardio exercise per week (Franklin et al., 2022).

On the other hand, resistance exercises, including weightlifting, bodyweight exercises like push-ups and squats, or the use of resistance bands, have demonstrated their efficacy in improving sleep by enhancing muscle strength and endurance. This reduction in discomfort and pain during the night contributes to overall sleep improvement. Beginners can initiate their journey into resistance training with bodyweight exercises, such as push-ups, squats, and planks. Begin with two to three sets of 10–12 repetitions of each exercise and progressively intensify the routine by incorporating weights or resistance bands as you advance (Kovacevic et al., 2018).

The practice of yoga, with its emphasis on stretching, controlled breathing, and mindfulness, has garnered recognition as a sleep-enhancing activity. Yoga's gentle stretches and poses release physical tension, while its controlled breathing techniques calm the mind, creating the ideal conditions for a peaceful night's sleep. Yoga is accessible to individuals of all fitness levels, making it an inclusive option for sleep improvement. Beginners can explore basic Hatha or gentle yoga classes, focusing on foundational poses and relaxation techniques, while those more experienced may opt for Vinyasa or Power Yoga for a more demanding practice. To reap the sleep benefits, consider incorporating yoga into your weekly routine (Bankar et al., 2013).

Breathing exercises, often integrated into yoga and meditation practices, offer remarkable tools for calming the mind and promoting relaxation. Techniques like deep diaphragmatic breathing or progressive muscle relaxation have been scientifically shown to alleviate stress and anxiety, two common contributors to sleep disturbances. Deep breathing exercises can be practiced virtually anywhere. Find a tranquil, comfortable spot to sit or lie down, close your eyes, and engage in deep breathing through your nose, holding the breath briefly, and then exhaling slowly through your mouth. Repeating this process for several minutes while focusing on your breath can effectively alleviate tension and prepare you for a restful night's sleep (Bankar et al., 2013).

Regular stretching routines, particularly before bedtime, release accumulated muscle tension, facilitating a more comfortable sleep posture. It's easy to incorporate stretching into your daily regimen —spend 10–15 minutes stretching major muscle groups after your morning shower or before bedtime, with special attention to areas prone to tension, such as the neck, shoulders, and lower back. Gentle stretches like neck tilts, shoulder rolls, and hamstring stretches can alleviate discomfort and prepare your body for a more relaxed slumber.

If you are just embarking on your fitness journey or have **age-related concerns**, gentle exercises can pave the way to improved sleep.

- **Gentle stretches:** Regardless of age, gentle stretches have proven to be a fantastic way to ease into exercise. Simple neck tilts, shoulder rolls, and hamstring stretches can be comfortably performed at home. Begin with 10–15 minutes of stretching each day, paying special attention to areas where tension accumulates.

- **Walking:** Walking stands out as one of the most accessible exercises, making it an ideal choice for beginners and seniors. Start with a 10–15-minute walk and gradually increase the duration as you become more comfortable with the activity. If possible, choose outdoor settings, such as nature trails, to maximize mental health benefits.

If **you have been regularly exercising** and wish to elevate your sleep-enhancing efforts, consider incorporating cardio and resistance training into your routine.

- **Cardio workouts:** Intermediate exercisers can explore activities like dancing, swimming, or cycling. These cardio workouts elevate heart rate and release endorphins, contributing to relaxation and enhanced sleep quality. Aim for at least 150 minutes of moderate-intensity cardio exercise per week.
- **Resistance training:** The inclusion of resistance training further enhances sleep quality by reducing the risk of discomfort or pain during the night. You can initiate resistance training with bodyweight exercises like push-ups and squats, gradually adding weights or resistance bands as your strength progresses.

Experienced exercisers have a wide array of options to optimize sleep through physical activity.

- **Yoga:** Trained people can explore more advanced forms of yoga, such as Vinyasa or Power Yoga, which offer both physical challenges and mindfulness benefits. Incorporating yoga into your routine at least a few times a week can maximize the sleep benefits.

- **High-intensity workouts:** For those who thrive on intense workouts, high-intensity interval training (HIIT) can be an excellent choice. However, it is advisable to complete such workouts earlier in the day to prevent overstimulation before bedtime.

Now that we have tailored exercise recommendations for different fitness levels and age groups, let's delve into the optimal timing of exercise for achieving the best sleep outcomes.

Exercise and Sleep: A Prescription for Timing and Type

- **Morning workouts**: Engage in strenuous activities like high-intensity interval training (HIIT) or running between 6 a.m. and 10 a.m. The circadian rhythm is in an active phase during these hours, allowing for optimized workout benefits without compromising sleep (Potter et al., 2016).
- **Afternoon exercise**: Moderate-intensity exercises like swimming or cycling should ideally be performed between 2 p.m. and 6 p.m. (Collier et al., 2014).
- **Evening wind-down**: After 8 p.m., focus on gentler activities like yoga or stretching to prepare your body for sleep.

Avoid rigorous exercise within 3 hours of bedtime. Doing so prolongs sleep initiation and reduces sleep efficiency.

The prescription outlined above should guide your exercise regimen for maximizing sleep benefits. Tailor both the type and timing of your exercise to meet your specific sleep goals. As we always recommend, consult your healthcare provider before starting any new exercise program, especially if you have pre-existing conditions.

As this science-backed exploration shows, exercise presents a potent tool for enhancing sleep quality, with options tailored to individuals of all fitness levels and ages.

PRACTICAL MEAL PLANNING FOR OPTIMAL SLEEP

As we've previously discussed, the relationship between diet and sleep is a close one. The foods and dietary choices you make have a profound impact not only on your overall health but also on the quality of your sleep. Choosing the right foods and planning your meals thoughtfully can significantly enhance your sleep patterns and, by extension, your well-being.

For optimal sleep and overall health, it's advisable to focus on a balanced and nutritious diet. Incorporating a variety of foods from different food groups is essential. This includes whole grains, lean proteins, healthy fats, and an abundance of fruits and vegetables. These foods provide essential nutrients, such as fiber, vitamins, and minerals, which support the body's functions, including those related to sleep.

Timing your meals can also play a crucial role in promoting better sleep. It's recommended to have your dinner a few hours before bedtime—at least three (O'Connor, 2023). This allows your body enough time to digest the meal, reducing the risk of discomfort and indigestion during the night. It's worth noting that large, heavy meals right before bedtime can be counterproductive, as your body's metabolism tends to slow down during sleep.

Let's explore some sample meal plans and templates that can help you plan your meals for optimal sleep. These plans are adaptable and can accommodate different dietary preferences. Remember, the goal is to provide your body with the right nutrients without overloading it, promoting restful sleep.

Vegetarian meal plan:

- **Breakfast***:* A hearty bowl of oatmeal topped with sliced bananas, chia seeds, and a drizzle of honey. Oats are a source of complex carbohydrates, which can promote the production of serotonin, a sleep-regulating hormone. Bananas contain tryptophan, an amino acid that aids in melatonin production.
- **Lunch***:* A colorful salad with mixed greens, cherry tomatoes, cucumbers, and chickpeas, dressed with olive oil and lemon juice. This salad provides a combination of fiber, vitamins, and minerals that support overall health and can contribute to better sleep.
- **Snack***:* Greek yogurt with a sprinkling of almonds and a handful of blueberries. Greek yogurt is a source of lean protein, while blueberries contain antioxidants that may help reduce oxidative stress and improve sleep quality.
- **Dinner***:* A flavorful stir-fry with tofu, broccoli, bell peppers, and brown rice. Tofu is a good source of protein, and brown rice is a complex carbohydrate that can help regulate blood sugar levels, promoting restful sleep.
- **Evening snack***:* A cup of chamomile tea with a small serving of mixed nuts. Chamomile tea is known for its calming properties, while nuts provide a source of healthy fats that can help maintain steady blood sugar levels during the night.

This meal plan incorporates foods rich in sleep-supporting nutrients like tryptophan, melatonin, and complex carbohydrates. It also offers a variety of textures and flavors, making it a satisfying choice for those following a vegetarian diet.

Gluten-free meal plan:

- **Breakfast***:* Scrambled eggs with sautéed spinach and gluten-free whole-grain toast. Eggs are a source of protein, and spinach provides essential nutrients like magnesium, which can contribute to better sleep.
- **Lunch***:* A quinoa and black bean salad with diced avocado, tomatoes, and a cilantro-lime vinaigrette. Quinoa is a gluten-free whole grain that offers a balance of protein and complex carbohydrates.
- **Snack***:* Sliced apples with almond butter. Apples contain fiber, while almond butter provides healthy fats and protein.
- **Dinner***:* Grilled chicken breast with a side of roasted sweet potatoes and steamed broccoli. Sweet potatoes are rich in complex carbohydrates and can help promote the production of serotonin.
- **Evening snack***:* A cup of caffeine-free herbal tea and a small serving of mixed berries. Herbal tea is a soothing choice, and berries contain antioxidants that can benefit sleep.

This plan provides a balanced combination of nutrients and flavors while minimizing the intake of potential sleep-disrupting ingredients like refined sugars and processed grains.

Omnivore meal plan:

- **Breakfast***:* A spinach and feta omelet served with a side of whole-grain toast. Spinach provides magnesium and feta contributes tryptophan, while whole-grain toast adds complex carbohydrates.

- **Lunch**: A grilled chicken and mixed greens salad with a balsamic vinaigrette dressing. Lean chicken breast offers protein, and the greens provide fiber and essential nutrients.
- **Snack**: A small serving of cottage cheese with pineapple chunks. Cottage cheese is a source of casein protein, which may aid in overnight muscle recovery.
- **Dinner**: Baked salmon with quinoa and steamed asparagus. Salmon is rich in omega-3 fatty acids, which can have anti-inflammatory properties and benefit sleep.
- **Evening snack**: A warm glass of milk with a dash of honey. Milk contains tryptophan and can promote relaxation and better sleep.

This plan combines a variety of foods to provide essential nutrients for sleep. It includes sources of magnesium, tryptophan, and omega-3 fatty acids, all of which can contribute to improved sleep quality.

Vegan meal plan:

- **Breakfast**: Overnight oats made with almond milk, topped with sliced bananas, and a sprinkle of chia seeds. Almonds and chia seeds offer magnesium and healthy fats, while oats provide complex carbohydrates.
- **Lunch**: A quinoa and black bean bowl with roasted vegetables and a tahini dressing. Quinoa and black beans supply protein and complex carbohydrates, while tahini adds healthy fats.
- **Snack**: Sliced cucumbers with hummus. Cucumbers are hydrating, and hummus provides protein and healthy fats.

- **Dinner***:* Baked tofu with brown rice and a side of sautéed kale. Tofu offers plant-based protein, while brown rice adds complex carbohydrates. Kale is rich in magnesium.
- **Evening snack:** A warm cup of herbal tea and a small serving of mixed berries. Herbal tea is calming, and berries contain antioxidants that can support sleep.

This plant-based meal plan focuses on nutrient-dense foods to promote better sleep. It includes ingredients rich in magnesium, tryptophan, and healthy fats while minimizing potential sleep-disrupting components often found in animal-based products.

Regardless of your consumption choices, all these meal plans aim to enhance sleep quality by offering a well-rounded array of nutrients. These plans provide essential vitamins and minerals like magnesium and tryptophan, known to play a role in sleep regulation, as we have discussed before. Additionally, they include complex carbohydrates for blood sugar balance lean proteins for muscle recovery, and amino acids such as tryptophan.

The inclusion of healthy fats in these meal plans supports satiety and helps maintain steady blood sugar levels during the night. By focusing on unprocessed, nutrient-dense foods, these meal plans reduce the intake of additives, sugars, and processed ingredients that can disrupt sleep.

The diversity of flavors, textures, and nutrients in these meal plans makes them appealing and adaptable to various dietary preferences. Whether you're an omnivore or follow a vegan lifestyle, these plans can help you achieve a restful night's sleep by providing the necessary nutrients at the right times.

HOLISTIC LIFESTYLE ADJUSTMENTS

As we wrap up this chapter, it's crucial to recognize that the quest for quality sleep isn't a solitary endeavor but is intricately linked to various facets of your daily life. Exercise and diet, for instance, aren't solely about physical health; they are key players in the realm of sleep improvement. Engaging in regular physical activity, particularly when strategically timed, can deepen the rejuvenating phases of your sleep and make the process of drifting off easier. In the same vein, a well-balanced diet featuring sleep-supporting nutrients directly influences the rhythm of your sleep cycles.

But it doesn't stop there. Stress management techniques and maintaining a consistent sleep schedule are equally vital components. These aren't isolated tasks but interdependent steps that collectively contribute to enhancing your sleep quality and overall well-being.

Feeling empowered? You should be. As you've navigated through this chapter, you've gained actionable insights grounded in scientific research to elevate your sleep quality. Yet, this is just the beginning. The upcoming chapters will provide a comprehensive roadmap, supported by scientific findings, to lead you on this multifaceted journey toward achieving restorative sleep. By making deliberate choices throughout your day, including what you consume, how you move, and how you manage stress, you're not just enhancing isolated aspects of your life; you're establishing the groundwork for rejuvenating nights and revitalizing days that lie ahead.

Help Others to Get to Dreamland

Just as one candle lights another and can light thousands of other candles, so one heart illuminates another heart and can illuminate thousands of other hearts.

— LEO TOLSTOY

Sleep resembles a tranquil stream that ideally carries us into the realm of dreams, but when that stream becomes turbulent, drifting into slumber becomes a challenge. We've all experienced those restless nights when tossing and turning feels more familiar than drifting into dreamland as if the sandman misplaced our address.

However, if you've navigated through the pages of *Hello Sleep, Goodnight Insomnia*, you've unearthed a treasure map to peaceful nights and energetic mornings. Within this book, we've meticulously packed science-backed secrets and actionable steps, all aimed at guiding you to the land of nod, where yawning is reserved for waking up, not for bedtime.

With just a few taps on your phone or clicks on your computer, you can extend a helping hand to a fellow weary soul in finding their way to this same treasure trove.

Could you spare a moment to share the gift of restful sleep? Think of it as tucking someone in with a heartfelt goodnight wish. Your review might be the soothing lullaby that someone desperately needs, whispering to them, *Hey, here's how to conquer those sleepless nights!*

If you're using Audible, tap the three dots in the top right of your device and select "Rate and Review." Leave a few thoughtful sentences about the book and assign it a star rating.

For Kindle or e-reader users, scroll to the bottom of the book and swipe up to prompt the review option.

In case these methods have changed, you can always visit the book's page on Amazon or your purchase platform and leave a review directly there.

For paperback enthusiasts, scan the QR code provided below to share your review:

We extend our heartfelt gratitude for sharing our work.

Wishing you peaceful slumbers,

Drs. Yasmine Elamir and William Grist.

CHAPTER 4

THE 7-STEP FRAMEWORK TO BETTER SLEEP, BETTER LIFE

Finish each day before you begin the next, and interpose a solid wall of sleep between the two. This you cannot do without temperance.

— RALPH WALDO EMERSON

Imagine sleep as a calm and peaceful sea, where the gentle waves of restfulness carry you to shores of rejuvenation each night. In this serene environment, one's mind and body find solace, and the symphony of dreams takes center stage. Yet, in the vast expanse of life, there often looms a storm: the relentless tempest of stress. This turbulent storm can whip the sea into a frenzy, disrupting the tranquility of sleep. In such times, we need a steadfast shelter, a guiding light to navigate the tempestuous waters of stress and find our way back to the shores of restful slumber.

This chapter, dear reader, serves as that shelter. It offers a seven-step framework to help you weather the storms of stress and improve your sleep. But before jumping in, we will explore the relationship between anxiety and insomnia for over-stress management solutions for insomnia, and mindfulness techniques. These will be the final stepping stones you will need to make the 7-step framework work seamlessly.

THE ANXIETY-INSOMNIA CYCLE

Anxiety and insomnia often go hand in hand, creating a complex and exhausting cycle that impacts mental well-being and sleep quality. Anxiety refers to a state of excessive uneasiness and apprehension, often accompanied by heightened physiological responses, such as increased heart rate and the release of adrenaline (American Psychological Association, 2021). This heightened state is our body's way of preparing for potential threats, priming us for action. However, when this state persists at bedtime, it can become a significant barrier to falling asleep.

Imagine going to bed with worries on your mind, whether they revolve around work, personal life, or any other concerns. When you're in bed, the absence of distractions allows your mind to focus solely on these worries. This physiological reaction is designed to help you face threats by increasing your alertness and physical readiness, making you either stronger (to fight) or faster (to flee).

This triggers physical changes like increased heart rate and the release of adrenaline. These changes can overstimulate your body, making it nearly impossible to drift into a peaceful slumber. To make matters worse, you may find it anxiety-provoking to fall asleep the next night, restarting the cycle once more.

This cycle can manifest as persistent worry, dread, or apprehension. Despite feeling physically exhausted from anxiety, you may find yourself ruminating—thinking deeply about the same concerns repeatedly—or, if this cycle has been happening for a long time worrying about sleeping itself.

The link between the two involves the corticotropin-releasing hormone system and the locus coeruleus-autonomic nervous system. Chronic and repeated stress can cause both systems to overact, leading to a maladaptive state of heightened arousal which can worsen both anxiety and insomnia (Staner, 2003).

Anxiety disorders are among the most prevalent mental disorders in the general population, affecting up to 25% of individuals at some point in their lives. It's estimated that approximately 50% to 70% of individuals with generalized anxiety disorder experience symptoms of insomnia. In fact, sleep disturbances are considered the second most common symptom of mental distress in the U.S. (Staner, 2003). The odds of developing an anxiety disorder are significantly higher in individuals who experience sleep disturbances, regardless of whether they suffer from insomnia or hypersomnia (Neckelmann et al., 2007).

The anxiety-insomnia cycle is a challenging and complex relationship that affects countless individuals. Breaking free from this cycle will be essential to restore your sleep. So, break these two up, and let's dive into stress management techniques.

STRESS MANAGEMENT TECHNIQUES FOR INSOMNIA

Managing stress, particularly in the setting of insomnia, is a challenging endeavor, to say the least. Honing these skills designed to combat stress during bedtime will be essential in regaining control over your sleep.

As we have previously addressed, the relationship between stress and sleeplessness is complex. Frequent stress can lead to persistent activation of your body's stress response, preventing it from returning to its baseline state. Luis F. Buenaver, a sleep expert from Johns Hopkins (n.d.), explains that individuals who are in pain, have worries, or are dealing with challenging life situations may experience elevated stress hormone levels in their bodies. A poor night's sleep can further contribute to this hormonal imbalance, preventing these stress hormones from breaking down and leaving you in a perpetual state of heightened stress (Hopkins Medicine, n.d.).

Stress management techniques for insomnia are valuable tools that can significantly improve the quality of your sleep. These are designed to address the root causes of stress and anxiety, making it easier to relax and fall asleep. Let's delve into some of these methods and explore how they interact with the sleep cycle to enhance it:

- **Deep breathing** techniques can be a game-changer when it comes to managing stress and improving sleep. The act of taking slow, deep breaths triggers the body's relaxation response, reducing the production of stress hormones. This, in turn, helps lower your heart rate and blood pressure, creating a more conducive environment for sleep. When you incorporate deep breathing into your bedtime routine, it can signal to your body that it's time to wind down and prepare for rest.
- **Meditative movement** practices like yoga or tai chi offer a dual benefit for those seeking better sleep. Not only do they help reduce stress, but they also promote physical relaxation and flexibility. Engaging in these gentle, flowing movements before bedtime can release tension in your

muscles and calm your mind. It's a fantastic way to connect your body and mind, preparing both for a restful night's sleep.

- **Progressive relaxation** is a technique that involves systematically tensing and then relaxing each muscle group in your body. By doing this, you become more aware of the physical sensations in your body and can release built-up tension. This method not only helps with stress management but also aids in physical relaxation, allowing you to ease into a state of calm that is conducive to sleep.

- **Biofeedback** is a valuable tool for understanding and managing the physical manifestations of stress. It involves monitoring physiological functions such as heart rate, muscle tension, and skin temperature to gain insights into your body's responses to stress. By learning to control these responses through biofeedback, you can effectively reduce stress and anxiety, making it easier to achieve a state of relaxation ideal for sleep.

- **Mindfulness** is a practice that involves staying fully present and engaged at the moment. This means letting go of worries about the past or future and focusing on the here and now. Mindfulness can be particularly useful for individuals struggling with racing thoughts at bedtime. By training your mind to stay in the present moment, you can reduce the mental chatter that often interferes with falling asleep.

- **Body scan** meditation is a technique that involves mentally scanning your body from head to toe, paying attention to any areas of tension or discomfort. By becoming aware of physical sensations and allowing them to release, you can ease physical and mental tension, making it easier to drift off to sleep.

- **Guided meditation** is a structured form of meditation where an instructor or recording leads you through a series of visualizations or relaxation exercises. This can be particularly helpful for individuals who struggle to relax on their own. Guided meditation provides a framework for achieving a state of relaxation that is conducive to sleep.

These techniques are versatile and can be incorporated into your daily routine to promote relaxation and reduce stress. Whether you choose deep breathing, meditative movement, progressive relaxation, biofeedback, mindfulness, body scan meditation, or guided meditation, the key is consistency. Regular practice will allow you to build the skills necessary to manage stress and enhance your sleep quality.

Here's a guided meditation for sleep that combines various stress management techniques. You can read and record this meditation to listen to before bedtime. This meditation will help you relax, unwind, and prepare your mind and body for a restful night's sleep:

Begin by finding a comfortable and quiet space where you won't be disturbed. You can either sit in a comfortable chair or lie down on your back. Close your eyes and take a few deep breaths to center yourself.

Let's start with some deep breathing. Inhale slowly through your nose for a count of four, allowing your abdomen to rise as you fill your lungs. Hold your breath for a count of four, and then exhale slowly through your mouth for a count of six. Feel the tension leaving your body with each exhalation. Continue this deep breathing for a few more breaths.

Now, shift your focus to your body. Starting from the top of your head, imagine a warm, soft light gently scanning down your body, like a soothing wave of relaxation. As this light passes through each part of your body, let go of any tension or stress. Visualize it melting away, leaving that area deeply relaxed.

Feel the warmth and relaxation in your forehead, then let it flow down to your eyes and cheeks. Allow your jaw to relax, parting your teeth slightly. Feel the relaxation move down to your neck and shoulders, releasing any tightness. Let it flow through your arms, elbows, and wrists, all the way to your fingertips.

Now, bring your awareness to your chest and heart. Imagine a sense of lightness and peace enveloping this area. Your breath is steady, and your heart is calm.

Continue to guide the warm, soft light down to your stomach, where any knots of tension are gently unraveled. Let it flow down through your hips and into your legs, easing any discomfort. Finally, let the relaxation reach your feet, allowing you to feel grounded and at peace.

As you focus on your breath, each inhale brings in a sense of tranquility, and each exhale releases any remaining stress or worry. Your breath is like the gentle waves of the ocean, lulling you into a state of deep relaxation.

Now, imagine a beautiful, serene garden. Picture yourself in this garden, surrounded by the soft sounds of nature. You're lying on a comfortable bed, nestled under a clear, starry sky. The air is warm and soothing, and a gentle breeze caresses your skin. You can hear the calming rustle of leaves and the distant chirping of crickets.

With each passing moment, you sink deeper into relaxation. You are safe and at peace in this tranquil garden. Your mind is clear, and your body is at ease.

As you lie there, allow any remaining thoughts or worries to gently drift away. Imagine them turning into delicate paper boats that float away on a peaceful stream, disappearing into the distance.

At this moment, there is nothing to do, nowhere to be, and no one to please. You are here, in this serene garden, fully present and at ease. Your body is heavy and relaxed, and your mind is calm.

As you drift off into a deep, restful sleep, know that you are safe, protected, and supported. Sweet dreams await you in the embrace of the night.

You can record this meditation and listen to it before bedtime to help you relax and prepare for a peaceful night's sleep. Feel free to customize it to your preferences, adding soothing background music or nature sounds for an even more immersive experience.

Here are six more templates of guided meditations for sleep, each designed to help you relax and improve your sleep quality. You can record these and use them on different nights of the week.

4-7-8 Technique

- Inhale through the nose for 4 seconds.
- Hold the breath for 7 seconds.
- Exhale through the mouth for 8 seconds.
- Repeat this pattern for four breath cycles. This technique is based on an ancient yogic technique called pranayama, which helps with breath control. Research indicates that controlled breathing like this can help reduce stress, improve mental well-being, and improve sleep quality (Balban et al., 2023).

Body scan meditation

- **Preparation**: Find a quiet space where you won't be disturbed for the next few minutes. Lie down on your back in a comfortable position—perhaps on your bed or a yoga mat. Close your eyes.

- **Focused attention**: Start by taking a few deep, diaphragmatic breaths. This activates the parasympathetic nervous system and initiates the body's relaxation response. Imagine the air you're breathing in is a warm, soothing light.
- **Head-to-toe scan**: Begin at the top of your head. Visualize this warm, soothing light moving slowly downward from your scalp through to your forehead and then to your facial muscles. As this light moves, consciously release tension in these areas.
- **Progressive relaxation**: Continue this downward scan from your neck, through your shoulders, arms, chest, and abdomen, all the way down to your toes. As you direct this warm light through each body part, take note of any tension or discomfort and allow it to dissipate.
- **Final release**: By the time this warm light has reached your toes, you should feel a sense of complete relaxation throughout your body. Let go of any residual tension.
- **Mindful awareness**: Take a moment to focus on your breath and the relaxed state of your body. Acknowledge the serenity that you have cultivated within yourself.
- **Completion**: Slowly open your eyes. Take a moment before standing up.

Guided visualization

- **Preparation**: Find a quiet and peaceful setting where you won't be interrupted for the next few minutes. Get into a comfortable position, either sitting or lying down, and close your eyes.
- **Induction**: Take a few deep, diaphragmatic breaths to begin the relaxation process. This engages the

parasympathetic nervous system and paves the way for relaxation.

- **Mental landscape**: Imagine a serene environment that makes you feel completely relaxed and at ease. This could be a beach, a forest, or any setting that brings you peace. The key is to involve all your senses—sight, sound, smell, and touch.

- **Engage the senses**: As you explore your serene environment, focus on the sensory details. If you're on a beach, feel the sand between your toes, hear the waves crashing, and smell the salt in the air—the more vivid your visualization is, the more effective your relaxation will be.

- **Deeper relaxation**: Allow this sensory experience to immerse you completely. Feel your body relaxing more deeply as you engage with your imagined environment. Your parasympathetic nervous system will become more activated, reducing cortisol levels and promoting relaxation.

- **Positive affirmations**: While in this relaxed state, you may opt to repeat some positive affirmations or mantras that resonate with you, further deepening your state of relaxation and reducing any lingering anxiety.

- **Gradual return**: As you prepare to exit your visualized environment, slowly start becoming aware of your physical surroundings. Feel the surface you're sitting or lying on, hear any ambient sounds, and when ready, gently open your eyes.

- **Grounding**: Before you stand up or move, take a moment to mentally scan your body and acknowledge the relaxed state you've achieved.

Mindfulness meditation

- Begin by taking a few deep, purposeful breaths. Inhale deeply through your nose, hold for a moment, and then exhale fully through your mouth. This acts as a "reset" for your nervous system and prepares your body for meditation.
- Turn your attention inward, specifically to your breathing. Observe each inhalation and exhalation without trying to modify them. Feel the air moving in and out of your nostrils or your chest rising and falling.
- It's natural for your mind to wander. When you notice that happening, don't chastise yourself. Acknowledge the stray thought and then gently steer your attention back to your breath. This act of acknowledging and refocusing is, in fact, a crucial part of the mindfulness practice.
- As you maintain your focus on your breath, begin to extend your awareness to other physical sensations. Feel the weight of your body against the chair or floor, notice any tension, and mentally release it with each exhale.
- If maintaining focus on your breath becomes challenging, you can use it as an "anchor" to return to when distractions occur. Each time your thoughts drift, think of your breath as an anchor that brings you back to the present.
- After a few minutes, or when you feel adequately relaxed and centered, start to become aware of your surroundings gradually. Hear the ambient sounds, sense the room's temperature, and slowly open your eyes when ready.
- Take a moment to assess how you feel. Do you feel more relaxed, less anxious, more in the present? Acknowledge these feelings, as they underscore the effectiveness of your practice.

Progressive muscle relaxation

- Lie down comfortably and close your eyes.
- Begin by tensing and then relaxing each muscle group in your body, starting with your toes and working your way up to your head.
- Focus on the release of tension with each relaxation.
- By the end, your entire body will be in a state of deep relaxation.

Biofeedback meditation

- Find a quiet space and close your eyes.
- Imagine a biofeedback machine that provides you with real-time information about your body's stress levels.
- As you focus on deepening your breath and releasing tension, visualize the readings on the biofeedback machine gradually lowering, reflecting a state of increasing calm and relaxation.

This meditation helps empower you with the ability to regulate your own stress responses by becoming more in tune with your body's physiological state.

These guided meditations can be recorded and used to help you unwind and prepare for a restful night's sleep. Use them on different nights of the week to create a soothing bedtime routine that promotes better sleep. Feel free to customize them to your preferences, adding background music or nature sounds for a more immersive experience.

Take the time to explore them by practicing and choosing the most suitable for you.

MINDFULNESS

Mindfulness is a powerful tool that can help you achieve deeper, more restful sleep. It involves being fully present in the moment, allowing you to be more aware of your thoughts and emotions without judgment. This practice can set the stage for restful slumber by helping you release anxieties that might keep you awake. The connection between mindfulness and sleep quality is profound, and here's why.

Dr. Shelby Harris, a clinical sleep psychologist, explains that many individuals dread the night and grow anxious about falling asleep, worrying that they won't be able to function the next day without sufficient rest (Mindful, 2020). This anxiety can create a cycle of stress that worsens sleep quality. However, mindfulness can break this cycle by increasing your awareness of thoughts and allowing you to let go of anxiety rather than becoming entangled in it. Strengthening your "mind muscle" through daily mindfulness practice helps you identify negative, insomnia-inducing thoughts and let them pass.

Mindfulness introspection readies your mind for sleep and can improve its quality. Studies have shown that mindfulness may be as effective as other highly recommended insomnia treatments (Rusch et al., 2018).

It's strongly recommended to practice mindfulness before sleeping to treat insomnia consistently. Below, you'll find some practical advice:

- If sleep eludes you, don't stay in bed awake for too long. Doing mindfulness practices outside of bed can help establish the association that the bed is primarily for sleeping. The goal isn't to fall asleep during your practice, but rather to ease your mind and then return to bed.

- Relying on sleep apps as a sedative is not ideal. It's best not to become dependent on external factors to fall asleep. You don't want to find yourself in a situation where your phone isn't available or the app doesn't work.
- Trying to force sleep when you're having trouble drifting off is often counterproductive. Accept the moment, acknowledge your concerns about sleep, and observe your busy mind. Visualize these thoughts floating away. The more you practice this acceptance and let go of the struggle, the easier it becomes to fall asleep.

Worries and stress are common culprits that rob us of sleep, keeping us awake as we replay concerns in our minds. Jared Minkel, a behavioral sleep expert, offers four strategies to use mindfulness to calm a worried mind and sleep more soundly (Bayes-Fleming, 2019):

- **Encourage positive distractions:** Instead of focusing on your inability to sleep, distract yourself with positive and engaging imagery that involves multiple senses or shift your focus. Picture a tranquil beach and immerse yourself in the sensory details: the sound of waves, the warmth of the sun, and the taste of salt. These mental images can eventually manifest in your dreams, so keep them pleasant and positive.
- **Allow worrisome thoughts:** If you're kept awake by stressful thoughts, don't try to push them away. Acknowledge that these thoughts are leading to emotions and these emotions are merely vibrations in the body that will eventually pass. Ride the wave and watch the

vibrations sail away. You will return to your normal life. Avoid replaying the worst scenarios repeatedly.

- **Practice nightly mindfulness:** Consistency is key to mindfulness for sleep. Regular practice will make you adept at directing your attention to the present moment instead of lying awake worrying about the future. Focus on your breathing or a physical sensation like the warmth and softness of your blankets. You can also try a body scan meditation to relax your body and mind.
- **Focus on gratitude:** Concentrating on positive aspects of your life can evoke pleasant emotions and help soothe you to sleep. Instead of dwelling on potential misfortunes, shift your attention to something or someone you're grateful for. Remember that your thoughts dictate your emotions. So, if you have positive thoughts, positive emotions and biological alterations will follow.

So, take the first step, explore mindfulness, and unlock the potential for more peaceful nights and brighter days.

SEVEN STEPS TO BETTER SLEEP

You've already analyzed the complexities of sleeping, exploring its vital connection to nutrition, physical health, aware consumption, stress, and mindfulness. Now, it's time to synthesize all that knowledge into a practical and simple 7-step guide. This guide is designed to provide you with a clear, actionable plan to significantly enhance your sleep quality. We'll summarize everything you've uncovered so far and present it in a straightforward step-by-step format. Each step represents a vital component in your pursuit of better sleep, and by following this program, you'll be well on your way to experiencing the rejuvenating power of restful slumber. Let's see it:

Step 1: Maintain a regular bedtime routine

Why: A consistent bedtime routine is like a lullaby for adults. It provides a signal to your body that it's time to relax and prepare for sleep. Our bodies have an internal body clock, known as the circadian rhythm, that helps regulate sleep-wake cycles. Disrupting this rhythm can lead to sleep problems. By sticking to a regular bedtime, you're training your body to recognize when it should be getting drowsy and when it should be alert.

Benefits: The benefits of a regular bedtime routine extend far beyond just getting a good night's sleep. It helps to establish a structured daily schedule, which can reduce stress and anxiety. This, in turn, leads to better sleep quality, with less time spent tossing and turning.

How: To maintain a regular bedtime routine, choose a fixed bedtime and wake-up time, even on weekends. Create a relaxing pre-sleep ritual, such as reading a book, taking a warm bath, or practicing deep breathing exercises. Avoid the temptation to disrupt your routine by staying up late or sleeping in; consistency is key.

Step 2: Control your environment

Why: Your sleep environment is the backdrop for your nightly slumber. It plays a critical role in determining the quality of your sleep. A comfortable and conducive environment can minimize disruptions and promote restful sleep.

Benefits: An optimized sleep environment allows you to fall asleep faster and enjoy deeper, uninterrupted sleep. This leads to improved cognitive function, mood, and overall well-being.

How: Start by ensuring your bedroom is dark, quiet, and cool. Invest in comfortable bedding, including a good mattress and pillows. If external noise is a concern, consider using white noise machines or earplugs. You may also want to dim the lights in your home as bedtime approaches, signaling to your body that it's time to wind down.

Step 3: Monitor food and drink

Why: What you consume can have a significant impact on your sleep. Certain foods and beverages can hinder your ability to fall asleep and stay asleep.

Benefits: Making conscious choices about what you eat and drink before bedtime can prevent discomfort, such as heartburn or indigestion, that might wake you up during the night. It also contributes to improved digestion and sleep efficiency.

How: Avoid heavy, rich, or spicy meals close to bedtime. These can lead to discomfort and indigestion. Caffeine and alcohol are known to sleep disruptors, so limit their consumption in the evening. If you're hungry before bed, choose light, easily digestible snacks like a banana, yogurt, or a small handful of nuts. Staying hydrated is important, but try to limit your fluid intake in the hours leading up to bedtime to reduce nighttime awakenings.

Step 4: Manage stress

Why: Unmanaged stress can lead to anxiety, making it difficult to relax and fall asleep. Stress management is essential for achieving a calm and peaceful state of mind.

Benefits: Practicing stress management techniques improves sleep quality by reducing nighttime anxiety and preventing insomnia. It's a pathway to a restful night's sleep.

How: Incorporate mindfulness, relaxation exercises, or meditation into your daily routine. These practices can help calm your mind before bedtime. Deep breathing exercises, progressive muscle relaxation, or mindfulness meditation can be particularly effective. By making stress management a regular part of your daily life, you'll create a foundation for better sleep.

Step 5: Avoid stimulants

Why: Stimulants like caffeine and nicotine can disrupt your body's natural sleep-wake cycle. They keep you awake and alert when you should be winding down.

Benefits: Reducing stimulants allows your body to prepare for sleep naturally. It leads to quicker and more restorative sleep, without the interruptions caused by these substances.

How: Limit your intake of caffeine and nicotine in the hours leading up to bedtime. Both substances can stay in your system for hours, affecting your sleep quality. Opt for caffeine-free herbal teas or warm milk as calming alternatives in the evening. By breaking the stimulant cycle, you'll improve your chances of falling asleep faster and staying asleep throughout the night.

Step 6: Regular physical activity

Why: Regular exercise has numerous benefits for sleep. It can reduce the time it takes to fall asleep and improve sleep quality.

Benefits: Engaging in regular physical activity promotes deeper sleep and reduces the number of nighttime awakenings. It's not only about better sleep but also enhanced mood and overall well-being.

How: Exercise regularly, but avoid intense workouts close to bedtime, as they can be stimulating. Aim to complete your more vigorous exercises at least three hours before bedtime. Gentle activities like stretching, yoga, or a leisurely walk are ideal closer to bedtime and can promote relaxation.

Step 7: Avoid screens before bedtime

Why: Screens emit blue light that can interfere with your body's internal clock and suppress melatonin production, the hormone responsible for regulating sleep.

Benefits: By avoiding screens the hour before bedtime, your body recognizes that it's time to wind down and prepare for sleep. This leads to quicker and more restful slumber.

How: Create a screen-free wind-down routine in the hour before bedtime. Instead of staring at a screen, engage in relaxing activities like reading a book, practicing relaxation exercises, or listening to calming music. The absence of screen-induced blue light ensures your body can naturally prepare for sleep.

By understanding the "why" behind each of these seven steps and applying the "how," you can significantly improve your sleep quality, leading to a more refreshed, alert, and vibrant you. Better sleep is within your reach by implementing these straightforward yet effective strategies.

The steps you've just learned are your path to a night of restful slumber, and the benefits will ripple through your days, making you more alert, focused, and ready to tackle life's challenges with newfound energy.

But this is just the beginning. In the bonus chapter, we'll delve even deeper into the secrets of a rejuvenating night's sleep. You'll discover additional tools, tips, and resources to enhance your sleep quality, providing you with an even brighter future filled with vitality and joy.

Your commitment to improving your sleep is a testament to your dedication to a healthier, happier life. The transformation has begun, and the best is yet to come. Get ready for the bonus chapter, where we'll unlock even more of the sleep-related treasures that await you.

Sweet dreams!

CONCLUSION

Each night, when I go to sleep, I die. And the next morning, when I wake up, I'm reborn.

— GANDHI

As we conclude this guide, the central message is clear and uncomplicated: You have within your grasp the tools for achieving better sleep and, by extension, a more fulfilling life. Through the seven carefully outlined steps presented in this book, you've been handed a science-backed blueprint. The efficacy of these steps isn't in mere understanding but in day-to-day application. Incorporate them into your routine to unlock tangible improvements in your mental sharpness, physical vitality, and overall emotional well-being.

By maintaining a regular bedtime routine, you are laying the foundation for consistent, rejuvenating sleep. It's about syncing your body's internal clock so that it knows when it's time to rest and when it's time to rise. Imagine the feeling of waking up each day refreshed and ready to conquer whatever challenges lie ahead. This step is the doorway to that dream.

Controlling your sleep environment is the second vital step. You've learned how lighting, temperature, and noise can significantly impact sleep quality. By taking charge of these elements, you are creating the optimal setting for restful sleep. As you adjust your environment, you'll notice that your nights are no longer interrupted by discomfort or disturbances. Instead, you'll experience a peaceful, uninterrupted slumber that leaves you recharged and ready to face a new day.

Monitoring your food and drink is the next essential step. You've delved into the world of nutrition, understanding how your diet can either promote or hinder your sleep. By making informed choices and developing a healthier relationship with food and drink, you'll discover that your nights are no longer plagued by digestive discomfort or blood sugar fluctuations. Instead, you'll find that your body and mind are at ease, allowing you to slip into a deep, restful sleep.

The fourth step is all about managing stress, which is the silent disruptor of our sleep. You've explored the intricate relationship between anxiety and insomnia and how one can spiral into the other. Incorporate stress management techniques, like mindfulness, into your daily life, and you'll find that your mind is calmer, your worries are less intrusive, and sleep becomes a more natural, peaceful part of your life.

The fifth step is a reminder to avoid stimulants. You've learned that substances like caffeine and alcohol can profoundly impact your sleep, often for the worse. By reducing or eliminating these stimulants from your life, you're ensuring that your sleep isn't disrupted by jittery nerves or restless nights. Instead, you'll be free to embrace the tranquility of sleep, night after night.

Step six emphasizes the importance of regular physical activity. Exercise isn't just about staying fit; it's also a fantastic stress reliever. You've seen how it can improve sleep quality, especially for those with insomnia. By incorporating regular physical activity into your life, you're not only improving your overall health but also enhancing your sleep.

The final step, avoiding screens before bedtime, is your gateway to a peaceful transition from wakefulness to slumber. You've learned about the detrimental effects of screen time before bed and how it can disrupt your sleep-wake cycle. By adopting a screen-free wind-down routine, you're allowing your mind to relax and prepare for a restful night's sleep.

In this book, you've explored these steps in detail, understanding why they matter and how to embrace them fully. Now, your journey to better sleep has begun, but remember that it's not just about reading these words; it's about living them. Embrace these steps, make them a part of your daily routine, and witness the profound changes they bring to your life.

As you reach the end of this book, remember that your commitment, patience, and consistency are the keys to unlocking the rejuvenating power of sleep. The journey has just begun, and the brighter future you've longed for is within reach.

And before you go, consider sharing your experience by leaving a review. Your words can guide others to the solution and practical advice they need for a better night's sleep. By helping others, you're contributing to a world where more people wake up revitalized and ready to seize the day. Your voice can be the beacon of hope someone is searching for.

Now, rest well and awaken to the life you've always dreamed of.

And... Cut!

BONUS CHAPTER: CBT WORKBOOK, SLEEP SUPPLEMENT GUIDE, AND 17 SHORT BORING BEDTIME STORIES

Welcome to the bonus section, a treasure trove of resources dedicated to improving your sleep. Inside, you'll discover a CBT workbook filled with insightful worksheets, a comprehensive sleep supplement guide, and a delightful collection of 17 short bedtime stories. These resources are tailored to complement your journey toward restful nights. With these tools in hand, you'll gain a deeper understanding of sleep science and find practical solutions for your unique sleep challenges. Let's dive in and unlock the secrets to your best night's sleep!

CBT WORKBOOK

Sleep Diary

One of the essential tools in CBT-I is maintaining a sleep diary. This powerful exercise will help you and your healthcare provider gain insight into your sleep patterns, identify areas for improvement, and tailor strategies to your unique needs (TalkPlus, n.d.).

Instructions:

1. Create a chart for each day of the week.
2. In the left column, write the days of the week (e.g., Monday, Tuesday, etc.).
3. In the next two columns, record the time you went to bed and the time you woke up. For example, if you went to bed at 11:00 p.m. and woke up at 7:00 a.m., you'd write "11:00 p.m." and "7:00 a.m." in the respective columns.
4. After a week of consistent tracking, review your sleep diary with a healthcare provider or use it as a reference to identify patterns and areas for improvement.

This sleep diary is a valuable tool in your journey to better sleep. It provides a visual representation of your sleep habits, which is crucial for recognizing patterns and understanding what might be contributing to your sleep challenges.

Sleep diary example:

Day	Time went to bed	Time woke up
Monday	11:00 p.m.	7:00 a.m.
Tuesday	10:30 p.m.	6:45 a.m.
Wednesday	11:15 p.m.	7:30 a.m.
Thursday	11:30 p.m.	6:15 a.m.
Friday	11:45 p.m.	7:15 a.m.
Saturday	12:00 a.m.	8:00 a.m.
Sunday	11:00 p.m.	7:30 a.m.

Empty sleep diary for you to fill:

Day	Time woke up
Monday	
Tuesday	
Wednesday	
Thursday	
Friday	
Saturday	
Sunday	

Use this empty sleep diary to record your sleep patterns for the next week. After a week of consistent tracking, you can review your diary for insights into your sleep habits and discuss potential improvements with a healthcare provider or use it as a reference as you work through the CBT-I techniques in this workbook.

Sleep Diary With Sleep Restriction

Sleep deprivation is a condition resulting from a consistent lack of sufficient sleep and can exacerbate insomnia problems by intensifying the difficulty in falling and staying asleep due to increased hyperarousal and heightened stress responses (TalkPlus, n.d.).

Sleep diary with sleep restriction template:

Day	Time went to bed	Time woke up	Time fell asleep	Time woke up	Time awake during the night	Time asleep	Time in bed	Sleep efficiency (%)	Sleep window
Monday									
Tuesday									
Wednesday									
Thursday									
Friday									
Saturday									
Sunday									

Instructions:

1. Each morning, fill out the sleep diary for the previous night.
2. Record the time you went to bed and the time you woke up in columns A and B.
3. In columns D and E, write down the time you fell asleep and the time you woke up.
4. In column F, estimate the total time you were awake during the night.
5. Calculate the average time asleep each night (in minutes) and record it in column G.
6. Calculate the average time in bed each night (in minutes) and record it in column C.
7. Calculate the sleep efficiency by dividing the total time asleep (column G) by the total time in bed (column C), then multiply by 100. Record it in column J.

8. Calculate the sleep window based on your average time asleep. If your sleep efficiency is below 80%, reduce the window by 15 minutes, but it cannot be less than 5 hours.
9. Set your sleep window and stick to it, even on weekends.

Example:

Day	Time went to bed	Time woke up	Time fell asleep	Time woke up	Time awake during the night	Time asleep	Time in bed	Sleep efficiency (%)	Sleep window
Monday	11:00 p.m.	7:00 a.m.	11:30 p.m.	6:30 a.m.	20 minutes	7 hours	8 hours	87.5%	7 hours
Tuesday	11:15 p.m.	6:45 a.m.	11:45 p.m.	6:30 a.m.	30 minutes	6 hours 45	7 hours 30	90.0%	6 hours 45
Wednesday	11:30 p.m.	7:15 a.m.	11:45 p.m.	7:00 a.m.	15 minutes	6 hours 45	7 hours 45	85.7%	6 hours 45
Thursday	11:00 p.m.	6:30 a.m.	11:30 p.m.	6:15 a.m.	45 minutes	6 hours 15	7 hours 15	86.2%	6 hours 15
Friday	10:45 p.m.	7:00 a.m.	11:15 p.m.	6:45 a.m.	30 minutes	7 hours	8 hours	87.5%	7 hours
Saturday	11:30 p.m.	7:15 a.m.	11:45 p.m.	7:00 a.m.	15 minutes	6 hours 45	7 hours 45	85.7%	6 hours 45
Sunday	11:00 p.m.	6:30 a.m.	11:30 p.m.	6:15 a.m.	45 minutes	6 hours 15	7 hours 15	86.2%	6 hours 15

Use this sleep diary with sleep restriction to monitor and manage your sleep patterns, gradually improving the quality and duration of your sleep. This technique can be a valuable part of your journey to conquer insomnia and improve sleep efficiency.

Insomnia Action Plan

Another important tool is using an insomnia action plan (Veteran Training, n.d.):

Write your answers on the line or check the appropriate boxes.

1. What emotional state, situation, or event led to poor sleep last time?

_____

_____

2. What emotional or situation can potentially hinder my sleep now?

_____

_____

Check the following ones:

- Negative emotional state: depression, stress, anxiety
- Positive emotional state: birth of child or grandchild, upcoming vacation, something exciting
- Illness: current illness or injury or an upcoming procedure that involves hospitalization or pain meds that may cause daytime sleeping
- Medical conditions: sleep apnea, thyroid dysfunction, chronic pain

3. Is there anything on the horizon that can impact my sleep?

Examples: Travel, new relationship, meeting.

_____

_____

4. Which parts of my new sleep routine helped me treat my insomnia the most?

☐ Keeping the same wake-up time every day (no matter how much sleep I get)
☐ Not trying too hard to sleep
☐ I go to bed when I'm sleepy but never before my regular bedtime
☐ Getting out of bed when I'm unable to sleep (20-minute rule)

5. Creating a buffer zone before bed

☐ Getting out of bed if I find myself worrying or having trouble stopping racing thoughts
☐ Engaging in worrying or problem-solving earlier in the evening
☐ Limiting the amount of time I spend in bed each night
☐ Using the bed for sleeping or sex only; removing items that may tempt me such as TVs, tablets, smartphones, etc.
☐ No napping (except for short safety naps)
☐ Not having caffeine or alcohol and not smoking cigarettes or engaging in strenuous exercise within a few hours of my bedtime

6. Write a specific reminder or statement about things you changed or techniques you used to help you cure your insomnia.

(Example: I always used to turn on the TV as soon as I got into bed, and I would lie there and watch hours of TV that kept me alert and awake. Removing the TV from my bedroom was the biggest and best change I made to help me cure insomnia. It also gives me a great sense of accomplishment that I did this on my own and cured my insomnia)

_____

_____

_____

_____

_____

_____

Things I need to remember at all times:

1. Don't compensate for sleep loss. If I have a bad night of sleep, don't "turn in early" the next night, stay in bed longer the next morning, or nap during the day.
2. Maintain my sleep schedule. Adjustments to the current sleep schedule should occur in 15-minute increments only and only on one side of the sleep schedule (i.e., morning or night, not both at the same time).
3. Never stay in bed awake for more than 20 minutes.
4. If insomnia starts and persists for more than a few days, keep a sleep diary and resume sleep prescription immediately.

You should review your action plan regularly and update it based on what is going on in your life.

How often would you realistically review and edit your action plan? Weekly, monthly, every two months?

_____

_____

Challenging Thoughts Worksheet

Also from Veteran Training (n.d.), the challenging thoughts worksheet:

Situation	Emotions (intensity %)	Automatic thought (belief %)	Evidence FOR	Evidence AGAINST	Balanced thought	Outcome
Describe the situation.	What emotions were you feeling?	Exactly what were you thinking when you felt these strong emotions? (How much do you believe this thought?)	What is the evidence that this thought is true?	What is the evidence that this thought is NOT true?	Re-write your original thought to consider ALL of the evidence (both for and against)	Did your emotions change? How much do you believe the original thought now
I can't fall asleep	*Frustration*	*I'll never fall asleep. Tomorrow will be miserable.*	*I'm awake now. I may not fall back asleep.*	*The dog has kept me awake before, and I fell back asleep. I haven't died from less than 8 hours of sleep.*	*Even though I'm awake, I'll be able to eventually fall back asleep, and I'll live without 8 hours of sleep.*	*You are able to fall back asleep.*

Situation	Emotions (intensity %)	Automatic thought (belief %)	Evidence FOR	Evidence AGAINST	Balanced thought	Outcome

Constructive Worry

While constructive worry can be beneficial, harmful worry tends to be counterproductive. Harmful worry is excessive, irrational, and often unrelenting. It's the type of worry that keeps you awake at night, running through endless worst-case scenarios without offering any meaningful solutions (Veteran Training, n.d.).

Harmful worry can take many forms, from ruminating about past mistakes to fearing unlikely future events. This type of worry doesn't lead to problem-solving; instead, it traps you in a cycle of anxiety and sleeplessness. It's like a hamster wheel for the mind, where you expend energy but get nowhere.

In contrast, constructive worry, when used appropriately, can have a more neutral or even positive impact on your sleep. When you engage in constructive worry, you're focused on solutions and planning rather than dwelling on problems. It's a purpose-driven process that allows your mind to work through challenges in a constructive manner, which can lead to feelings of accomplishment and reduced stress.

The following chart can help you to illustrate better the correct approach to deal with these concerns:

What am I worried about?	Is this something that I can control?	What can I do to address this concern?
Upcoming job interview	*Yes*	*Research the company, prepare answers to common interview questions, and practice my presentation skills.*
Health of a loved one	*Partially (can offer support)*	*Check in with them, offer assistance, and encourage them to seek medical advice if necessary.*

Stimulus Control

Below are the behaviors you may need to modify in order to be successful in treating insomnia (Veteran Training, n.d.).

Limit your activities in bed to just sleep and sex: What activities are you currently doing in bed that you need to stop? Examples include eating in bed, playing with your smartphone, and watching TV.

Don't get into bed until you are sleepy:

What does sleepy mean?

- I can barely keep my eyes open.
- I keep nodding off.
- I keep yawning.

What does tired mean?

- I'm mentally exhausted from that meeting today.
- I'm worn out from the gym today.

Get out of bed if you are unable to fall asleep within 20 minutes: What activities can you do if you don't fall asleep within 20 minutes of going to bed? Examples include making a to-do list, light stretching, or folding laundry.

Eliminate napping: How does napping impact your sleep needs? What activities can you do to keep you from napping? Examples include taking a short walk, doing a chore, or walking the dog.

NOTE: If you feel sleepy and have to operate a vehicle or machinery or perform any activity where your or someone else's safety is in danger, take a nap.

Progressive Relaxation Worksheet

Progressive muscle relaxation is a technique aimed at achieving a state of physical and mental calmness. The primary objective of this method is to induce a serene physical and mental state, ultimately aiding in the initiation of sleep. Its origins can be traced back to the pioneering work of Dr. Edmund Jacobson, who introduced this technique in 1908 and subsequently detailed its procedure (Jacobson, 1924).

The progressive muscle relaxation exercise involves several steps:

1. Recognize even the slightest muscular tension within the body.
2. Assess each muscle group for tightness, commencing with the larger muscle groups.
3. Gradually relax each muscle group, often by initially tensing the muscles tightly and then fully releasing the tension.
4. As a new muscle group is relaxed, the individual should maintain relaxation in all previously relaxed muscles, creating a cumulative effect.
5. Continue this process of muscle group relaxation until complete relaxation is attained, embodying the essence of progressive muscle relaxation.

Once individuals become adept at achieving full relaxation, they may bypass the step-by-step muscle group approach and proceed directly to complete relaxation. It is worth noting that mastering the skills required for progressive and full relaxation necessitates dedication, time, and consistent practice.

Here's an example of the order for progressive muscle relaxation:

- Right foot
- Left foot + right foot
- Right calf + left foot + right foot
- Left calf + right calf + left foot + right foot
- Right upper leg + left calf + right calf + left foot + right foot

- Left upper leg + right upper leg + left calf + right calf + left foot + right foot
- Hips + entire right leg + entire left leg + feet
- Low back + hips + legs + feet
- Mid back + low back + hips + legs + feet
- Upper back + mid back + low back + hips + legs + feet
- Shoulders + entire back + hips + legs + feet
- Right hand + shoulders + back + hips + legs + feet
- Left hand + right hand + shoulders + back + hips + legs + feet
- Right arm + left hand + right hand + shoulders + back + hips + legs + feet
- Left arm + right arm + hands + shoulders + back + hips + legs + feet
- Chest + arms + hands + shoulders + back + hips + legs + feet
- Neck (front and back) + entire upper body + entire lower body
- Face (including the jaw to the forehead) + neck + upper body + lower body
- Scalp + face + neck + upper body + lower body
- Complete relaxation of every muscle in the body simultaneously

If each muscle group is given 15–30 seconds for relaxation, the entire process will typically last for about 5–10 minutes. Additionally, individuals can enhance the experience by first adding tension to the muscles before relaxation, such as wiggling the toes and then relaxing them, stretching the legs and then relaxing, and so on. Listening to soothing music, applying a warm compress to the targeted muscles, practicing deep breathing, and focusing on the sensation of muscles becoming progressively heavier and sinking into the bed can further elevate the effectiveness of this technique (Free CBT-I, n.d.).

What is the goal of progressive relaxation?

_____

What are the steps for progressive muscle relaxation?

_____

What does it take to learn how to be skilled at progressive muscle relaxation?

_____

What is the order of muscles you would like to use in your progressive muscle relaxation?

_____

Are you open to using progressive muscle relaxation?

_____

What are your thoughts on using progressive muscle relaxation every night for 1 week, 2 weeks, 1 month?

_____

A List of Activities

Use the table below to list down activities that can

- help you relax your body and your mind and help you go back to sleep if you were to wake up in your sleep window.
- lead to a heightened emotional or physical arousal, which eventually disrupts your sleep quality and chances of going back to a sound sleep.

Keep this list somewhere so it is easily visible to you. Add or remove activities as you test them out throughout your treatment process (Rossman, 2019).

Activities conducive to good sleep	Activities that can worsen my sleep
Reading a book	Scrolling on social media

Thought Record

A thought record is a cognitive-behavioral tool that helps individuals identify and challenge negative or irrational thoughts. It's commonly used in CBT to improve mental health and manage conditions like anxiety and depression. By keeping a thought record, you can gain insight into your thought patterns, recognize distorted thinking, and work toward more balanced and constructive thoughts (Rossman, 2019).

- **Date and time:** [Insert date and time of the thought]
- **Situation or trigger:** Describe the situation or event that prompted your thought.
- **Emotions (rate intensity %):** List the emotions you're experiencing, and rate their intensity from 0% (not intense) to 100% (extremely intense).
- **Automatic thought (AT):** Write down the thought that immediately came to mind in response to the situation.
- **Evidence supporting AT:** List any evidence that supports your automatic thought.
- **Evidence against AT:** Identify any evidence that contradicts or weakens your automatic thought.
- **Balanced or alternative thought (BT):** Generate a more balanced, rational, or constructive thought that considers the evidence both for and against your initial automatic thought.
- **Emotions after challenging AT (rate intensity %):** Reassess your emotions after working through the thought, and rate their intensity.

You can use the following chart to fill in:

	Monday	Tuesday	Wednesday	Thursday	Friday	Saturday	Sunday
Date and time	5th March						
Situation/ trigger	A job meeting the next morning						
Emotions (%)	Anxiety, stress, worry						
Automatic thought	*I won't sleep enough and I'll mess it up tomorrow*						
Evidence for AT	Lack of sleep drives bad mood and inefficiency						
Evidence against	*I have been in this situation before and I have managed to handle it*						
Balanced thought	*I will relax so I can sleep and be ready for the meeting*						
Emotions after AT	Calm						

Passive Wakefulness

Passive wakefulness, often employed by individuals who experience difficulty falling asleep due to anxiety about sleeplessness, serves as a highly effective technique. Instead of remaining in bed while plagued by the distress of insomnia, this approach encourages individuals to deliberately attempt to stay awake. By redirecting their focus toward the antithetical goal of staying awake, they can gradually release their anxieties and, in turn, facilitate a smoother transition into slumber (Troxel et al., 2012). This method provides an insightful strategy for managing sleep-related apprehensions, ultimately promoting a more restful night's sleep.

A Trip to Hypnagogia

The process of falling asleep entails traversing a transitional state known as hypnagogia, characterized by the presence of hallucinogenic "dream fragments" rather than complete dreams, which typically emerge around 50 minutes after the initial onset of sleep (Troxel et al., 2012). Self-hypnosis is a technique that actively encourages and beckons the hypnagogic phase, a state often devoid of conscious recollection. An age-old strategy that shares a similar purpose is the mental exercise of counting sheep, which, although laborious, stimulates imagery within the mind and potentially initiates the journey into hypnagogia.

In Megan's case, We introduced her to self-hypnosis techniques that not only fostered the hypnagogic state but also induced relaxation. Megan quickly became proficient in employing these techniques independently. Additionally, she found solace in utilizing the visualizations we practiced, mirroring those used in our sleep sessions, to promote restful slumber. For instance, guiding clients to visualize mundane activities can gently lead them into the realm of hypnagogia.

Over time, the positive outcomes were evident as Megan regained her ability to sleep through the night. She described her transformation as akin to rebirth, reclaiming the happiness that had been robbed from her by the clutches of sleeplessness.

It's important to note that not all techniques and approaches mentioned here are universally applicable to every client. However, We trust that you've found valuable insights in this discussion that can be tailored to your specific therapeutic context.

SLEEP SUPPLEMENT GUIDE

Are sleep supplements the answer to your restless nights? It's a question many find themselves pondering in the wee hours of the night. Sleeplessness can be incredibly frustrating, leading some to consider the use of sleep supplements. However, it's vital to approach this topic with caution and responsibility. Let's delve into a comprehensive guide on sleep supplements, their advantages, drawbacks, and the best practices for their use.

Sleep supplements come in various forms, from over-the-counter options to prescription medications. They are designed to help you fall asleep more easily or stay asleep throughout the night. While these can be short-term solutions for specific sleep-related challenges, it's essential to recognize their limitations. Incorporating these antihistamines into your sleep routine should be a well-considered decision. They are typically used for short-term relief from sleep difficulties and are best suited for occasional use rather than as a long-term solution. Consulting with a healthcare professional is advisable before starting any regimen, especially if you have underlying health conditions or are taking other medications.

Melatonin

Routine use of melatonin may not be ideal due to its potential to shift circadian rhythms. However, this property can be advantageous for shift workers who can strategically use melatonin to adjust their sleep patterns when working overnight, improving sleep quality and adaptation to new schedules (Turek & Gillette, 2004). For someone working overnight shifts on Monday, Wednesday, and Sunday, she could strategically use melatonin supplements. On her work nights (Monday and Wednesday), she might take melatonin before bedtime to improve sleep during the day. However, on non-work nights (Tuesday, Thursday, Friday, and Saturday), she should avoid melatonin to allow her circadian rhythms to adjust naturally and promote regular nighttime sleep.

Dosing guidelines:

- Start with 0.5–1 mg: Begin with a low dose, typically between 0.5–1 mg, about 30 minutes to an hour before bedtime.
- Adjust as needed: Depending on your response, you can gradually increase the dose, but it's generally recommended not to exceed 3–5 mg.

How to use:

- Time it right: Take melatonin about 30 minutes before your intended bedtime.
- Consistency: Use it consistently to help regulate your sleep-wake cycle.

Pros:

- Faster sleep onset: Melatonin can aid in falling asleep more quickly.
- Minimal side effects: It generally has few side effects when used as directed.
- Non-habit forming: Melatonin is non-addictive and can be used without concerns about dependence.

Cons:

- Potential drowsiness: Some users may experience grogginess the following day.
- Not effective for everyone: It doesn't work for everyone, and its effectiveness may vary from person to person.

Valerian Root

Dosing guidelines:

- Start with 300–600 mg: Commence with a dose of 300–600 mg, usually 30 minutes to two hours before bedtime.
- Adjust gradually: Adjust the dose as needed, but avoid exceeding 1200 mg per day.

How to use:

- Allow time: Give valerian root sufficient time to take effect before heading to bed.
- Regular use: Consistent use may provide the best results.

Pros:

- Improved sleep quality: Valerian root may enhance sleep quality and reduce the time it takes to fall asleep.
- Non-addictive: It's non-habit forming and generally safe for short-term use.

Cons:

- Gastrointestinal issues: Some individuals may experience stomach discomfort.
- Not suitable for long-term use: It's best used as an occasional aid and not recommended for extended periods.

L-Theanine

Dosing guidelines:

- Typical dose: A common dose ranges from 200–400 mg about an hour before bedtime.

How to use:

- Pair with caffeine: L-Theanine may be used in combination with caffeine during the day to reduce its stimulating effects.

Pros:

- Relaxation: L-Theanine promotes relaxation and may help reduce anxiety, facilitating better sleep.
- No daytime drowsiness: It usually doesn't cause drowsiness during the day.

Cons:

- Effectiveness variability: Its effectiveness can vary from person to person.
- Limited sedative effect: L-Theanine is not a strong sedative, so it may not be suitable for severe insomnia.

Tryptophan

Dosing guidelines:

- Typical dose: Start with 500–1000 mg, preferably taken with a light carbohydrate snack, about 30 minutes to an hour before bedtime.
- Adjust as needed: Depending on your response, you can increase the dose up to 2000 mg.

How to use:

- Pair with carbohydrates: Tryptophan is more effective when consumed with carbohydrates, as it helps with its absorption into the brain.
- Consistency: Consistent use is essential to observe its effects on sleep.

Pros:

- A precursor to melatonin and serotonin: Tryptophan is a precursor to both melatonin and serotonin, which play key roles in regulating sleep.
- Low risk of dependency: It is generally not habit-forming and is considered safe when used appropriately.

Cons:

- Slow onset: It may take some time to notice its effects, and it's not suitable for those looking for immediate sleep assistance.
- Individual variability: Its effectiveness may vary from person to person.

5-HTP (5-Hydroxytryptophan)

Dosing guidelines:

- Typical dose: Begin with 50–100 mg, taken 30 minutes to an hour before bedtime.
- Gradual increases: Depending on your response, you can gradually increase the dose but avoid exceeding 300 mg per day.

How to use:

- Avoid mixing with MAOIs: Do not use 5-HTP if you are taking MAOI antidepressants.
- Consistency: Consistent use may provide better results.

Pros:

- A precursor to serotonin: 5-HTP is a precursor to serotonin, which influences sleep patterns.
- May improve mood: It may also have a positive effect on mood, potentially reducing anxiety or depression-related sleep disturbances.

Cons:

- Potential nausea: Some users may experience mild gastrointestinal discomfort, particularly at higher doses.
- Interactions: It can interact with certain medications, so consult with a healthcare provider before use.

Passion Flower

Dosing guidelines:

- Typical dose: Start with 400–500 mg, taken about an hour before bedtime.
- Adjust as needed: Depending on your response, you can increase the dose but avoid excessive amounts.

How to use:

- Regular use: Consistency is key for experiencing the potential benefits of passion flower.

Pros:

- Sedative properties: Passion flower has mild sedative properties that may promote relaxation and improve sleep.
- Non-addictive: It's typically non-habit forming and considered safe for short-term use.

Cons:

- Effectiveness variability: As with many supplements, its effectiveness can vary from person to person.
- Not for severe insomnia: It's best suited for mild to moderate sleep disturbances.

Chamomile tea

Dosing guidelines:

- Typical dose: Steep 1–2 teaspoons of dried chamomile flowers in hot water for about 5 minutes. Or enjoy your favorite brand-name pre-packaged tea.
- Frequency: Enjoy a cup of chamomile tea 30 minutes to an hour before bedtime.

How to use:

- Consistency: Consistent use is key to experiencing its potential sleep-inducing effects.
- Avoid heavy meals: Enjoy it on an empty or lightly filled stomach for best results.

Pros:

- Natural sedative: Chamomile is a natural sedative that can help promote relaxation and reduce anxiety, making it a suitable sleep aid.
- No side effects: Unlike medications, chamomile tea doesn't carry the risk of side effects like daytime drowsiness or dependence.

- Potential anxiety relief: Some individuals find it can be more calming than Xanax, a prescription medication known for its anti-anxiety effects.

Cons:

- Effectiveness variability: As with any natural remedy, individual responses to chamomile tea may vary.
- Not immediate: Its effects may not be as rapid as pharmaceutical sleep aids, so it's important to allow time for its calming influence.

Ashwagandha

Dosing guidelines:

- The recommended dose of Ashwagandha for sleep support typically falls in the range of 300–500 mg.

How to use:

- To reap potential sleep benefits, maintain a consistent Ashwagandha regimen.
- Different forms of Ashwagandha are available, such as powder, tea, pills, tinctures, or gummies. Follow the specific instructions provided on the product you choose.
- It is advisable not to use Ashwagandha continuously for more than three months. Regularly consult with your healthcare provider during its use.

Pros:

- Promoting relaxation: Ashwagandha may help reduce stress and anxiety, common culprits of sleep disturbances. Its potential to promote relaxation can indirectly lead to better sleep.
- Improved sleep quality: Preliminary research suggests that Ashwagandha may aid in faster sleep onset, prolonged sleep duration, and overall enhanced sleep quality.
- Non-addictive: Unlike some sleep medications, Ashwagandha is generally considered non-addictive and does not carry the risk of dependency.

Cons:

- Individual variability: Responses to Ashwagandha can vary among individuals, and its effectiveness for sleep may be influenced by various factors.
- Not immediate: It's important to note that the effects of Ashwagandha on sleep may not be immediate, and patience may be required.
- Side effects: Mild side effects of Ashwagandha may include diarrhea, nausea, upset stomach, vomiting, dry mouth, drowsiness, vertigo, hallucinations, cough, congestion, blurred vision, rash, or weight gain.
- Liver damage: There is some evidence suggesting that Ashwagandha supplements might pose a risk of liver damage. If you encounter symptoms consistent with liver issues, such as jaundice or itchy skin, consult your healthcare provider immediately.

Cannabidiol, commonly known as CBD, is a natural compound derived from the cannabis plant. It has gained popularity for its potential health benefits, including sleep improvement. CBD comes in different forms, and two primary variants are full spectrum and broad spectrum. Let's explore them in detail.

Full Spectrum CBD

Full-spectrum CBD contains a wide range of cannabinoids, including tetrahydrocannabinol (THC). THC is the psychoactive compound in cannabis responsible for the "high" sensation. Due to the presence of THC, full-spectrum CBD will negatively affect the sleep and wake cycles and even lead to weight gain, which can be undesirable for those seeking restful sleep. WE RECOMMEND AVOIDING!

Broad Spectrum CBD

In contrast, broad-spectrum CBD offers the potential benefits of cannabinoids without the inclusion of THC. This absence of THC makes broad-spectrum CBD a preferred choice for individuals aiming to manage sleep without the psychoactive effects associated with THC.

Benefits:

Recent studies and articles have shed light on how broad-spectrum CBD may contribute to better sleep:

- Anxiety reduction: Some individuals find broad-spectrum CBD helpful in managing anxiety, a common disruptor of sleep patterns. Research indicates that CBD may have anxiolytic (anxiety-reducing) effects, promoting relaxation conducive to sleep.

- Pain management: Pain can be a significant impediment to quality sleep. Studies suggest that CBD's anti-inflammatory properties may help alleviate pain, potentially enhancing sleep quality.
- Stress reduction: Chronic stress can disrupt sleep patterns. Broad-spectrum CBD's potential to reduce stress may indirectly contribute to improved sleep.

Hot to use:

When considering broad-spectrum CBD for sleep, it's essential to follow guidelines to ensure safety and effectiveness:

- Consultation with healthcare providers: Prior to starting any CBD regimen, consult with your healthcare provider, especially if you have underlying health conditions or are taking medications that may interact with CBD.
- Dosage considerations: Start with a low dosage, typically around 10–20 mg, and gradually increase as needed. Personalized dosing is crucial as CBD's effects vary among individuals.

CBD is available in various forms, including oils, capsules, gummies, and topicals. Here's how to use it effectively:

- Oil or tinctures: Place a few drops under your tongue, hold for about 30 seconds, and then swallow. Effects may take about 30 minutes to an hour to kick in.
- Capsules: Swallow capsules with water. Effects may take longer to appear, usually within 1–2 hours.

- Gummies: Chew and swallow gummies. They may take about 30 minutes to an hour to take effect.

Pros:

- Potential for anxiety reduction.
- Potential for pain relief.
- Potential for stress reduction.
- Non-psychoactive, no "high" associated with THC.

Cons:

- Limited regulation in the CBD market leads to variations in product quality.
- Potential mild side effects, including dry mouth, dizziness, and changes in appetite.

Side effects:

While CBD is generally well-tolerated, some individuals may experience mild side effects like dry mouth, dizziness, or changes in appetite. Monitoring and adjusting your dosage can help manage these effects.

While sleep supplements can offer temporary relief, they are just that, a temporary solution to a bigger problem. However, they do have a short-term role while working on the skills needed to restore your sleep and vitality!

Magnesium

Magnesium is a mineral that plays a crucial role in various bodily functions. It is important to follow proper dosing guidelines when considering magnesium supplementation. Here are some dosing guidelines, instructions on how to use it, as well as the pros and cons associated with magnesium supplementation.

Dosing guidelines:

- The recommended daily allowance (RDA) for magnesium varies depending on age and gender. For adult males, the RDA is around 400–420 mg, while for adult females, it is around 310–320 mg.
- It is advisable to consult with a healthcare professional to determine the appropriate dosage for your specific needs.

How to use:

- Magnesium supplements are available in various forms, including capsules, tablets, powders, and liquids.
- Follow the instructions provided by the manufacturer or as directed by your healthcare professional.
- It is generally recommended to take magnesium supplements with food to enhance absorption and minimize the risk of digestive discomfort.

Pros:

- Magnesium supplementation may help support healthy bone density and strength.
- It plays a vital role in muscle function and can aid in muscle relaxation and recovery.

- Magnesium is involved in over 300 enzymatic reactions in the body, contributing to various physiological processes, including the sleeping cycle.

Cons:

- High doses of magnesium supplements may cause gastrointestinal side effects such as diarrhea, nausea, and abdominal cramps.
- Individuals with kidney problems or certain medical conditions should exercise caution and consult with a healthcare professional before taking magnesium supplements.

Glycine

This amino acid can help improve sleep by reducing sugar in the blood and fostering melatonin segregation and muscle relaxation.

Dosing guidelines:

- To improve sleeping quality, glycerin dose is typically between 3–5 grams taken orally.

How to use:

- You can get supplements of glycine in the form of powder or pills. Preferably, combine with solid light food rich in natural fats, like nuts or avocado, in your last meal of the day.

Pros:

- Reduces fatigue and drowsiness.
- It fosters quicker deep sleep.

Cons:

- Glycine is generally well tolerated by healthy adults. Side effects are uncommon, but may include nausea, vomiting, or mild stomach upset.

Inositol

Inositol is a naturally occurring compound that belongs to the vitamin B family. It is commonly used as a dietary supplement and is available in various forms, including capsules, powders, and tablets.

Dosing guidelines:

- The recommended dosage of inositol can vary depending on the specific health condition being treated. It is important to follow the instructions provided by your healthcare provider or the product label. Generally, the typical dosage ranges from 500–2000 mg per day, divided into multiple doses.

How to use:

- It can be taken with or without food, as directed by your healthcare provider. It is usually recommended to start with a lower dosage and gradually increase it if needed. It is important to follow the recommended dosage and not exceed the maximum daily limit.

Pros:

- It may help improve symptoms associated with polycystic ovary syndrome (PCOS), such as irregular menstrual cycles and insulin resistance.
- It helps regulate blood sugar levels, which can be beneficial for individuals with diabetes or metabolic syndrome.

Cons:

- In some cases, inositol supplementation may cause gastrointestinal discomfort, such as nausea, bloating, or diarrhea. These side effects are usually mild and temporary.
- Inositol may interact with certain medications, such as lithium and selective serotonin reuptake inhibitors (SSRIs). It is important to consult with your healthcare provider before starting inositol supplementation if you are taking any medications.

It's crucial to note that the effectiveness of these supplements can vary from person to person. If you're considering using any of these supplements, it's advisable to consult with a healthcare professional before incorporating them into your routine, especially if you have underlying health conditions or are taking medications, to ensure they are safe and suitable for your specific needs.

In addition to dosages and administration times, understanding potential side effects, drug interactions, and the appropriate duration for using these supplements is equally important for making an informed decision regarding their use.

SHORT BORING BEDTIME STORIES

The following stories are not designed to ignite your imagination or stir your emotions. Instead, they invite you on a tranquil journey into monotonous narratives, where gentle imagery and straightforward plots converge to create a sense of calm.

These narratives are crafted with a deliberate lack of excitement, and you might wonder why. In medical terms, you can think of these stories as a form of benign cognitive distraction—a gentle and uneventful diversion.

Their purpose is to divert your mind from the stresses and worries that often hinder your ability to fall asleep. By doing so, they create space for your natural sleep mechanisms to take over. In a way, it's akin to watching paint dry; in this case, the paint is the story itself, and as it dries, your eyelids naturally become heavy.

To make the most of these stories, integrate them into your bedtime routine right before bed. As you listen to or read these narratives, allow their monotonous themes to wash over you. Let your mind drift, embrace the soothing repetition, and feel the gentle currents of monotony guide you toward peaceful sleep. Now, enjoy... But not too much because that would defeat the purpose.

Story #1: The Mild Adventures of a Postal Worker

Our protagonist, John, is your everyday postal worker. He awakens precisely when the alarm clock insists, an old, reliable clock that faithfully does its job without any frills. He plods into the bathroom, where the toothbrush neither boasts of novelty nor decrepitude. It's just a toothbrush, and he uses it to scrub away sleep's remnants.

After the mundane morning ritual, John embarks on the short journey to the post office. His car is ordinary, a vessel of predictability that gets him there without a hiccup. At the post office, he diligently organizes the mail. Letters go into one slot, packages go into another, and the monotony of this task goes unchallenged.

As he steps into his delivery van, John takes to the roads, which, much like his toothbrush, are neither new nor old but entirely reliable. Traffic lights greet him, persistently green, offering no dramatic moments, just a continuous flow of the unremarkable.

Throughout the day, John delivers mail and packages, each destination more unexceptional than the last. He leaves a magazine through a mail slot, the very essence of a slot, on a door that's just a door and leaves packages on porches that don't demand a second glance.

When the sun hangs lower in the sky, John returns to the post office. He completes his day's work and says customary goodbyes to coworkers who possess a level of nondescript that rivals his own. After this uneventful day, he reflects for a moment, acknowledging that it was much like every other day—without any peaks or valleys, just a flatline of activity.

Story #2: How to Sort Socks

The first step in this sock-sorting saga is to assess the color. With a keen eye, the Sock Sorter scrutinizes each sock, seeking out its color twin. This is a matter of utmost importance in the world of socks. A black sock must meet another black sock, a white sock must find its partner in white, and so on. It's a systematic operation devoid of spontaneity.

Once the color code is deciphered, the Sock Sorter proceeds to examine the texture. Some socks are ribbed, while others are smooth, but the difference is more of a fact than a fascinating topic of discussion. These texture variations are noted, not celebrated.

The matching process continues in this manner: a meticulous pairing of socks, color by color, texture by texture. There is no room for improvisation or deviation from the established procedure. Each pair is formed with the same methodical approach, as if a machine designed to sort socks, devoid of any hint of excitement.

The sock-sorting odyssey concludes with rows of neatly matched sock pairs lying unassumingly in their designated drawer, ready to serve their utilitarian purpose. It's not an adventure but a task completed with precision and predictability.

Story #3: A Day in the Life of a Goldfish

Fin is a goldfish.

The day starts as it always does, with a splash of morning sunshine, barely illuminating the confines of a glass fishbowl. In this modest aquatic world, there's nothing grand or awe-inspiring, just endless laps around the bowl. Fin swims around in an eternal loop, a feat that might seem impressive but is, in reality, unceasingly dull.

At mealtime, which is a single event on this fishy calendar, Fin receives a single pinch of fish flakes. It's a portion that would barely fill a spoon for a human but suffices for our watery protagonist.

The afternoon is marked by yet another swim as if there could be any variation in this repetitive existence. As Fin glides through the water, a brief distraction ensues when the owner walks by. But this momentary excitement quickly dissipates, and the goldfish returns to its familiar loop.

The evening swim offers no surprises. The sun sets outside the window, casting dim reflections on the water's surface. And, just like that, the day ends. Fin finds a spot near a plastic plant, a plant that's neither real nor fake, and settles in for a night of restful, uneventful slumber.

Story #4: How to Water Indoor Plants

Watering indoor plants is an everyday task that we'll discuss in painstaking detail. The first step is selecting a rather unremarkable watering can, chosen for its functionality rather than its appearance.

Following this, we'll engage in the excitement of checking soil moisture. Using the finger-insertion method, we determine whether the soil is neither too wet nor too dry.

Now, onto the water-pouring spectacle. Lift the watering can, place its spout near the base of the plant, and pour water onto the soil. It's a slow and uneventful process, akin to watching paint dry. The water is absorbed by the soil with minimal fuss.

Story #5: Waiting for a Bus in Real-Time

At the bus stop, we stand in patient anticipation, the scene so typically unremarkable it could easily go unnoticed. We become one with the bus stop's lackluster surroundings, blending into the daily urban landscape.

The journey begins as we check our watch. The minute hand moves with the exquisite slowness of a glacier, a testament to the remarkable power of time when you're watching it.

Minutes two and three pass—just and our eyes catch a fleeting glimpse of a passing car. Its paint is unremarkable, and it moves neither too fast nor too slow—just a car passing by like countless others.

Minutes four and five are filled with action as we delve into reading a bus schedule. We examine it with unwavering focus, parsing through the precise timing of our impending ride.

Minutes six and seven mark a subtle shift in our demeanor. Slight impatience creeps in, just like the afternoon sun casting a longer shadow. We glance at our watch again, even though the minute hand has barely budged.

Finally, minutes eight through ten arrive with all the grandeur of a sudden downpour on a gloomy day. The bus pulls up to the stop, its doors hissing open. With a sense of satisfaction that can only be likened to finishing a lukewarm cup of tea, we board the bus and continue our journey to the end.

Story #6: How to Assemble a Basic Puzzle

To assemble a 100-piece puzzle depicting a cloudless sky, one should approach the task with a methodical and systematic approach. Begin by selecting a well-lit, flat surface as your workspace. This will provide adequate visibility and stability during the assembly process.

Sort the puzzle pieces into manageable groups. Categorize them based on distinct patterns or colors. For a cloudless sky puzzle, you might consider organizing pieces according to the varying shades of blue or any patterns that might be present, such as gradients or subtle differences in hue.

Start with the edge pieces. These are typically straight-edged and form the puzzle's perimeter. Assemble the edge pieces to create the puzzle's framework. Refer to the image on the box for guidance, as it will serve as your reference throughout the assembly.

Once the border is complete, focus on connecting pieces based on their color and pattern. Gradually build the puzzle by attaching pieces that fit together logically. Proceed methodically, ensuring that each piece interlocks with its neighbors.

Patience is key during this process. Expect to encounter moments of monotony and repetition, given the uniformity of a cloudless sky. Continue to match pieces according to their visual cues, and the image will gradually take shape.

As you near completion, the remaining pieces will become easier to place. Double-check your work, ensuring that all pieces fit precisely. Once the final piece is in position, step back and admire your completed puzzle of the cloudless sky, a testament to your meticulous and patient approach.

Story #7: The Journey of a Recycled Bottle

It all begins when the bottle meets its fate in the recycling bin, joining a pile of discarded containers destined for a second life.

From the recycling bin, our unremarkable plastic bottle embarks on its journey to a recycling facility. Here, it mingles with a sea of fellow containers, sorted and separated. The bottle's plastic companions are subjected to rigorous scrutiny, a tedious process that involves separating them by type, color, and quality. The facility's sorting machines function mechanically, exhibiting a dispassionate efficiency that mirrors the bottle's own unremarkable existence.

Once sorted, the bottle is next subjected to the thorough cleansing it desperately needs. Immersed in water, it's cleansed of the residue of its previous contents, and any lingering labels or glue are removed in a monotonous assembly-line operation. The water used for this task is recycled, aligning with the sustainability ethos that governs the recycling process.

Following its bath, the bottle is shredded into smaller pieces. The machinery responsible for this step operates with mechanical precision, reducing the bottle to tiny fragments. It's a process devoid of drama or flair, focused solely on preparing the plastic for its transformation into something new.

In the furnace of the recycling facility, our bottle, now in its shredded form, is melted down. The heat-driven liquefaction of the plastic is a straightforward and energy-intensive process devoid of fanfare. The molten plastic is then molded into new items, items that might find usefulness as part of a park bench or another unremarkable yet functional object.

In the end, the recycled plastic bottle, once a mundane part of our consumer existence, has transitioned into a new role as a park bench or some other equally prosaic entity. Its journey, devoid of any grandeur or excitement, underscores the practical, unglamorous reality of recycling and its role in sustainability, silently contributing to a circular economy.

Story #8: How to Reorganize a Bookshelf Alphabetically

Here's a detailed guide to help you achieve an orderly bookshelf arrangement:

Begin by clearing the bookshelf entirely. This blank canvas will make it easier to see what you're working with and avoid any confusion.

Next, gather all your books and place them in a single, manageable pile. Sorting them in a pile allows you to easily assess their titles and authors.

Now, let's address the question of "A" and "An." In alphabetizing book titles, these articles are generally ignored. For example, "A Tale of Two Cities" would be treated as if it were titled "Tale of Two Cities." This is a common practice in library and bookshop organizations, designed to simplify the process.

Arrange the books based on the first letter of the remaining words in their titles. For example, "The Great Gatsby" would be sorted under "G" for "Great." If two titles have the same starting letter, move on to the second letter, and so on, until they can be distinguished.

Now, consider the author's last name. If you're arranging your books by author, this step is crucial. In cases where multiple books share the same title and the author's name is the same, distinguishing between them can be challenging. In such situations, adding the publication year or edition number can help create a clear hierarchy.

For book series, keep all volumes together, either by title or author. For example, if you have a series of *Harry Potter* books, arrange them in order of the series, which might mean *Harry Potter and the Sorcerer's Stone* comes before *Harry Potter and the Chamber of Secrets*.

Avoid the temptation to group books by size or color. Alphabetizing should take precedence over aesthetic considerations.

Once your books are neatly arranged, step back and admire your organized bookshelf. It's a gratifying feeling to have your collection neatly accessible and ready for exploration.

Story #9: A 24-hr Surveillance Tape

In the security room of a nondescript building, the day begins with the quiet hum of surveillance equipment. The monitor displays an uneventful room, but the operator knows that, over the course of the next 24 hours, every minor event captured by the security tape will be recorded, regardless of its significance.

Morning arrives, and as the sun's gentle rays touch the exterior camera, the screen comes to life with images of birds. The mundane yet mesmerizing scene unfolds as avian visitors flit and flutter, seemingly oblivious to the watchful lens. It's a serene start to the day, a natural spectacle that reminds the operator of the world outside.

As the clock moves into the afternoon, the security tape records a passing car. It's an ordinary event, nothing more than a fleeting moment in the grand scheme of things. But to the surveillance tape, it's a record of life going on, people coming and going, each vehicle leaving a trace of its presence.

Evening descends, and the streetlights flicker to life, casting a warm, artificial glow on the otherwise dim street. The camera diligently captures this transition from day to night, from natural to artificial illumination. It's a routine occurrence, but the security tape faithfully documents it, a sentinel of routine events.

The night hours roll in, and there, under the streetlight's steady gaze, a stray cat appears. It prowls—an enigmatic figure in the dark, its movements cautious yet confident. The surveillance tape bears witness to the feline's presence, capturing a small, living being in the tapestry of ordinary occurrences.

As the clock nears the end of its cycle, the surveillance tape completes its 24-hour journey. The operator, with a sense of finality, presses the rewind button. The tape winds back, replaying the sequence of mundane yet somehow comforting events that transpired within its scope.

In the security room, the operator takes a moment to appreciate the uneventful day recorded by the surveillance tape. While it's easy to overlook the ordinary, this tape reminds us that even the most minor occurrences have their place in the narrative of existence. It's a story that unfolds every day, waiting to be captured by the watchful eyes of security cameras, preserving the subtle, fleeting moments that define our daily lives.

Story #10: How to Iron a Shirt

Begin by setting up your ironing board and iron in a well-lit and spacious area.

Lay the shirt flat on the ironing board, ensuring that it's straight and symmetrical. The shirt's front should face up, and the collar should be properly aligned.

Start with the collar. Gently stretch it out flat, making sure there are no creases or folds. Slowly move the iron over the collar from one end to the other, pressing out any wrinkles. Ensure the collar is crisp and smooth.

Moving to the shoulders, lay one side of the shirt on the ironing board, extending it fully. Iron the shoulder area, paying attention to any wrinkles or folds, and then switch to the other shoulder, repeating the process.

Now, focus on the sleeves. Begin with one sleeve and lay it flat on the ironing board, aligning the seams. Iron from the shoulder down to the cuff, taking care to eliminate any creases or wrinkles. Then, repeat the process for the other sleeve.

For the shirt's front and back, start with one side. Ensure the placket (the part with buttons or snaps) is properly aligned. Glide the iron in a straight line from the top down to the hem, pressing out any wrinkles. Rotate the shirt and continue ironing until the entire front side is smooth and wrinkle-free.

Repeat the same process for the other side of the shirt, maintaining the same meticulous approach to ensure a uniformly ironed garment.

Finally, iron the yoke, the area across the shoulders on the back of the shirt, paying close attention to any wrinkles or folds.

Inspect the entire shirt for any remaining wrinkles, paying special attention to the seams and corners. Touch up any problem areas as needed.

Once you've thoroughly ironed the entire shirt, hang it or lay it flat to cool and set the fabric. This helps to maintain the smooth appearance you've achieved.

Ironing a shirt requires patience and attention to detail, ensuring that each section is properly pressed, resulting in a well-groomed and wrinkle-free garment.

Story #11: The Quiet Neighborhood

As the story begins, the peaceful scene of this neighborhood is set. The sun rises, casting a gentle glow over the houses and tree-lined streets. It's a place where time seems to stand still, and the residents savor the serenity that envelops them.

Morning arrives, and the hush of the neighborhood remains undisturbed. But then, a solitary dog barks once, shattering the stillness for a brief moment. It's an unusual occurrence in this serene enclave, a lone voice that adds a touch of unpredictability to the otherwise tranquil morning.

The afternoon brings with it the predictable rhythm of life. A mail delivery person makes their rounds, placing letters and packages in mailboxes with practiced efficiency. It's a simple act, but it serves as a reminder that life quietly carries on, even in the most peaceful corners of the world.

Evening approaches and the sky takes on hues of soft pastels as the day gently transitions into night. A passing car hums along the residential street. It's a fleeting presence, a whisper in the otherwise hushed neighborhood, a reminder that the outside world occasionally intrudes.

With the arrival of night, the streetlights cast their warm, welcoming glow. They illuminate the streets and sidewalks, providing a sense of security in the quiet darkness. The neighborhood's nocturnal guardians stand as silent sentinels against the night's mysteries.

As the story concludes, the neighborhood returns to its peaceful slumber. The quiet envelops everything once more, and the simple sounds of the occasional dog bark or passing car serve as gentle reminders of life's subtle presence in this tranquil haven. In the quiet neighborhood, it's the uneventful days that are cherished, where the absence of commotion is the greatest gift.

Story #12: How to Make Instant Oatmeal

To prepare instant oatmeal, follow this detailed guide that covers boiling water, stirring in oats, and waiting until they reach an edible temperature without the use of lists:

Begin by selecting your preferred flavor of instant oatmeal. Choices vary from plain oats to flavored options like maple and brown sugar or apple cinnamon. Ensure you have a microwave-safe bowl or a heatproof container on hand.

Measure the appropriate amount of water for your oatmeal. This is typically between 1/2–1 cup of water per packet, depending on your preferred consistency. Pour the water into a microwave-safe container.

Place the container in the microwave and set the cooking time to approximately 1–2 minutes. The precise time may vary depending on your microwave's power. The goal is to bring the water to a rolling boil. Watch it carefully to prevent overflow.

Once the water is boiling, carefully remove the container from the microwave using oven mitts or a towel to avoid burns.

Open the instant oatmeal packet and pour the contents into the hot water. Stir the oats thoroughly to ensure they are well combined with the hot liquid.

Cover the container with a microwave-safe lid or a microwave-safe plate to trap the heat. This step is essential as it allows the oats to absorb the hot water and soften. Let the oatmeal sit for about 2-3 minutes.

After the waiting period, carefully uncover the container and stir the oatmeal again. This helps distribute any remaining hot spots and ensures a consistent texture.

Allow the oatmeal to sit for an additional 1-2 minutes or until it reaches a temperature that is safe to eat. Be cautious, as the oatmeal may still be very hot, and it's best to let it cool slightly before taking a bite.

Your instant oatmeal is now ready to enjoy. If you prefer, you can add extra toppings such as fresh fruits, nuts, or a drizzle of honey to enhance the flavor.

Story #13: Paint Drying

Watching paint dry on a wall may not be the most riveting activity, but it offers insight into the transformation of a freshly painted surface. We start with a wall that has just received a fresh coat of paint. At this stage, the surface is notably wet and exhibits a noticeable sheen, a far cry from the eventual matte finish.

As time passes, we observe a gradual reduction in wetness. The moisture present in the paint begins to evaporate, causing the surface to lose its initial glossiness. This marks the initial stages of the paint-drying process.

During the subsequent drying phase, there's a subtle alteration in hue. The colors deepen slightly as the paint settles and dries. This change is a result of the solvents in the paint evaporating, revealing the true, more saturated colors beneath.

In the final stage, the paint's surface becomes touch-dry and assumes a matte finish. This signifies the paint's complete drying process.

Ultimately, we are left with drywall, the outcome of a methodical and necessary process in creating a stable and appealing painted surface.

Story #14: Changing a Light Bulb

Changing a light bulb involves several steps that are easy to follow. The first and most critical step is to ensure your safety. Always turn off the power to the light fixture before attempting to replace the bulb. You can do this by either switching off the circuit breaker or unscrewing the current light bulb. Safety should never be compromised during this task.

Once you've ensured safety, it's essential to select the correct replacement bulb. Check the wattage and type of the old bulb, and find a new one that matches these specifications. Using the wrong type or wattage can lead to issues or even damage.

Before attempting to unscrew the old bulb, allow it to cool down if it has been on recently. Hot bulbs can be dangerous to touch and may shatter upon contact. Take your time and be cautious throughout the process.

Remove any lampshades or covers that might be blocking access to the bulb. In some fixtures, there might be a protective cover that needs to be gently taken off. Handle these parts with care, as they can be delicate.

When it's time to remove the old bulb, gently turn it counterclockwise. If it feels stuck, avoid using excessive force, as this can cause the bulb to break. To improve your grip, consider using a cloth or gloves.

Take a moment to clean the fixture if it's dirty or dusty. Dust and debris can affect the quality of the lighting, so a quick cleaning can make a noticeable difference.

Installing the new bulb is a straightforward process. Screw it in a clockwise direction, but take care not to overtighten it, as this can damage the fixture or the bulb itself.

With the new bulb securely in place, turn the power back on to test if the light is functioning correctly. If the light doesn't turn on, double-check that the bulb is firmly screwed in, and ensure that the circuit breaker is on.

Finally, if you removed any lampshades or covers, make sure to put them back in their original positions. Also, consider the responsible disposal of the old bulb, which may involve recycling or properly wrapping it in newspaper or a plastic bag before disposal.

Story #15: Watching Grass Grow

The growth of grass is a rather uneventful yet dependable process. It all starts with small seeds resting in the soil, quietly absorbing the necessary nutrients without any fuss. Gradually, tiny green shoots emerge from the ground, reaching skyward in a predictable, almost monotone fashion.

These young sprouts, not known for their enthusiasm, slowly stretch upwards, day by day, as if they were on an uneventful mission to touch the sun. At the same time, below the surface, the roots extend themselves methodically, not in a hurry, securing the grass firmly in its place in the earth.

As weeks turn into months, this unassuming grass becomes a soft, even carpet that covers the ground. It's as if it's programmed to be as uniform and predictable as possible, offering a rather plain but soothing presence to anyone who happens to observe it.

And so, the grass keeps growing with an unwavering determination. There's no rush, no excitement; it just follows its innate, almost hypnotic rhythm. If you were to watch it for a while, you'd probably find yourself drifting into a state of calm, much like the grass itself.

Story #16: Packing a Lunch

Packing a simple lunch involves several steps to ensure it's organized and enjoyable. Start by selecting an appropriate lunch container. This container should have compartments or be spacious enough to accommodate your sandwich, snacks, and any additional items.

For your sandwich, lay out your ingredients. Begin with two slices of bread. On one slice, evenly spread your preferred condiments, making sure not to make the bread soggy. Next, add your choice of protein, whether it's deli meat, cheese, or a plant-based option— layer on your desired vegetables, such as lettuce, tomatoes, and cucumbers. Finish by placing the second slice of bread on top, condiment side down to prevent sogginess. If you prefer, cut the sandwich in half.

Consider your snack choices to complement the sandwich. This could include fresh fruit like apple slices or grapes, and a portion of vegetables, such as carrot sticks or cherry tomatoes. Don't forget a small container of hummus or dipping sauce for added flavor. You might also include a handful of nuts or a granola bar for a satisfying addition.

Organize your sandwich and snacks within the lunch container. To prevent the sandwich from becoming soggy, you can use a separate small container for the condiments and add them to your sandwich just before eating.

Include any extras you enjoy, such as a small dessert, a piece of chocolate, or a drink. Place these items inside the lunch container, ensuring they are well-secured to prevent spillage.

If your lunch contains perishable items like dairy or mayonnaise, store it in the refrigerator until you're ready to eat. In cases where refrigeration isn't possible, use an insulated lunch bag with ice packs to keep your lunch fresh.

Before you head out, double-check that your lunch container is securely closed and that any necessary utensils or napkins are included. This comprehensive approach to packing your lunch ensures that it's well-prepared and organized, ready to be enjoyed at your convenience.

Story #17: The Silent Symphony

In a grand concert hall, the stage is set for a performance that never unfolds. The orchestral members arrive, a sea of musicians, each taking their place with precision and solemnity.

First, the violins take center stage. The musicians delicately tighten their bowstrings, and the room fills with the soft, high-pitched hum of strings being tuned. The delicate balance between tension and tone is a crucial element in crafting the perfect melody.

As the violins find their pitch, the woodwinds join in, each player taking care to ensure their reeds are properly fitted and adjusted. The woodwinds, with their flutes, clarinets, and oboes, bring a diverse range of harmonies to the silent symphony, each note resonating in perfect unity.

In the background, the percussion section is hard at work. Drummers meticulously test the drums and cymbals, ensuring that each strike will produce the intended timbre. The resonance of a well-struck drumhead vibrates through the air, adding to the anticipation of a performance that will never come.

Finally, the conductor arrives, a figure of authority and artistry. He raises his baton and, for a moment, there's a collective intake of breath in the concert hall. But then, the conductor lowers his arm, and the performance that was never meant to start remains suspended in silence.

The audience, expectant and eager, waits indefinitely. Each seat is filled with anticipation, the air humming with the latent potential of the musicians on stage. The hall itself seems to hold its breath as the silent symphony lingers in the air, a masterpiece that will never be played.

REFERENCES

Abernathy, K., Chandler, L. J., & Woodward, J. J. (2010). ALCOHOL AND THE PREFRONTAL CORTEX. *International Review of Neurobiology, 91*, 289–320. https://doi.org/10.1016/S0074-7742(10)91009-X

Alasmari, F. (2020). Caffeine induces neurobehavioral effects through modulating neurotransmitters. *Saudi Pharmaceutical Journal, 28*(4), 445–451. https://doi.org/10.1016/j.jsps.2020.02.005

American Academy of Sleep Medicine. (2015). *Practice guidelines.* American Academy of Sleep Medicine – Association for Sleep Clinicians and Researchers. https://aasm.org/clinical-resources/practice-standards/practice-guidelines/

American College of Physicians. (2016, May 3). *ACP recommends cognitive behavioral therapy as initial treatment for chronic insomnia.* acponline. https://www.acponline.org/acp-newsroom/acp-recommends-cognitive-behavioral-therapy-as-initial-treatment-forchronic-insomnia

American Psychological Association. (2021). Anxiety. *Https://Www.apa.org.* https://www.apa.org/topics/anxiety#:

Baglioni, C., Nanovska, S., Regen, W., Spiegelhalder, K., Feige, B., Nissen, C., Reynolds, C. F., & Riemann, D. (2016). Sleep and mental disorders: A meta-analysis of polysomnographic research. *Psychological Bulletin, 142*(9), 969–990. https://doi.org/10.1037/bul0000053

Balban, M. Y., Neri, E., Kogon, M. M., Weed, L., Nouriani, B., Jo, B., Holl, G., Zeitzer, J. M., Spiegel, D., & Huberman, A. D. (2023). Brief structured respiration practices enhance mood and reduce physiological arousal. *Cell Reports Medicine, 4*(1). https://doi.org/10.1016/j.xcrm.2022.100895

Bankar, M. A., Chaudhari, S. K., & Chaudhari, K. D. (2013). Impact of long term Yoga practice on sleep quality and quality of life in the elderly. *Journal of Ayurveda and Integrative Medicine, 4*(1), 28. https://doi.org/10.4103/0975-9476.109548

Bayes-Fleming, N. (2019, March 15). *What to do when worry keeps you awake.* Mindful. https://www.mindful.org/what-to-do-when-worry-keeps-you-awake/

Bhaskar, S., Hemavathy, D., & Prasad, S. (2016). Prevalence of chronic insomnia in adult patients and its correlation with medical comorbidities. *Journal of Family*

Medicine and Primary Care, 5(4), 780–784. https://doi.org/10.4103/2249-4863. 201153

Binks, H., E. Vincent, G., Gupta, C., Irwin, C., & Khalesi, S. (2020). Effects of diet on Sleep: A narrative review. *Nutrients, 12*(4), 936. https://doi.org/10.3390/nu12040936

Blume, C., Garbazza, C., & Spitschan, M. (2019). Effects of light on human circadian rhythms, sleep and mood. *Somnologie : Schlafforschung Und Schlafmedizin = Somnology : Sleep Research and Sleep Medicine, 23*(3), 147–156. https://doi.org/10.1007/s11818-019-00215-x

Brainly Quotes. (n.d.). *Leonardo da Vinci Quotes.* BrainyQuote. https://www.brainyquote.com/quotes/leonardo_da_vinci_154282

~~Brainly Quotes~~Steinbeck, J. (n.d.). *John steinbeck quotes.* BrainyQuote. https://www.brainyquote.com/quotes/john_steinbeck_103825

Brainy Quotes. (n.d.). *John Steinbeck Quotes.* BrainyQuote. https://www.brainyquote.com/quotes/john_steinbeck_103825

Brower, K. J. (2001). Alcohol's effects on sleep in alcoholics. *Alcohol Research & Health, 25*(2), 110–125. https://www.ncbi.nlm.nih.gov/pmc/articles/PMC2778757/

Cappuccio, F. P., D'Elia, L., Strazzullo, P., & Miller, M. A. (2010, May 1). *Sleep duration and all-cause mortality: A systematic review and meta-analysis of prospective studies.* Sleep. https://pubmed.ncbi.nlm.nih.gov/20469800/

CBT Denver. (n.d.). *Cognitive Behavioral Therapy for Insomnia (CBT-I) — CBT Denver.* CBT Denver. https://www.cbtdenver.com/treatment-approaches/cognitive-behavioral-therapy-for-insomnia-cbt-i

CDC. (2020, April 28). *Health effects of smoking and tobacco use.* Centers for Disease Control and Prevention. https://www.cdc.gov/tobacco/basic_information/health_effects/index.htm#:

Chaput, J.-P., Dutil, C., Featherstone, R., Ross, R., Giangregorio, L., Saunders, T. J., Janssen, I., Poitras, V. J., Kho, M. E., Ross-White, A., Zankar, S., & Carrier, J. (2020). Sleep timing, sleep consistency, and health in adults: a systematic review. *Applied Physiology, Nutrition, and Metabolism, 45*(10 (Suppl. 2)), S232–S247. https://doi.org/10.1139/apnm-2020-0032

Collier, S., Fairbrother, K., Cartner, B., Alley, J., Curry, C., Dickinson, D., & Morris, D. (2014). Effects of exercise timing on sleep architecture and nocturnal blood pressure in prehypertensives. *Vascular Health and Risk Management*, 691. https://doi.org/10.2147/vhrm.s73688

Colten, H. R., & Altevogt, B. M. (2006). *Extent and health consequences of chronic sleep loss and sleep disorders.* Nih.gov; National Academies Press (US). https://www.ncbi.nlm.nih.gov/books/NBK19961/

Daviet, R., Aydogan, G., Jagannathan, K., Spilka, N., Koellinger, P. D., Kranzler, H.

R., Nave, G., & Wetherill, R. R. (2022). Associations between alcohol consumption and gray and white matter volumes in the UK Biobank. *Nature Communications, 13*(1). https://doi.org/10.1038/s41467-022-28735-5

Dickens, C. (2020). *Bleak House*. Alma Classics.

Fernandez-Mendoza, J., & Vgontzas, A. N. (2013). Insomnia and Its Impact on Physical and Mental Health. *Current Psychiatry Reports, 15*(12), 418. https://doi.org/10.1007/s11920-013-0418-8

Fiorentino, L., & Martin, J. L. (2010). Awake at 4 a.m.: Treatment of Insomnia With Early Morning Awakenings Among Older Adults. *Journal of Clinical Psychology, 66*(11), 1161–1174. https://doi.org/10.1002/jclp.20734

Franklin, B. A., Eijsvogels, T. M. H., Pandey, A., Quindry, J., & Toth, P. P. (2022). PHYSICAL ACTIVITY, CARDIORESPIRATORY FITNESS, AND CARDIOVASCULAR HEALTH: A clinical practice statement of the American Society for Preventive Cardiology Part I: Bioenergetics, contemporary physical activity recommendations, benefits, risks, extreme exercise regimens, potential maladaptations. *American Journal of Preventive Cardiology*, 100424. https://doi.org/10.1016/j.ajpc.2022.100424

Free CBT-I. (n.d.). *CBTi Everything On One Page and Printable PDF*. Free Cognitive Behavioral Therapy for Insomnia, CBTi. http://freecbti.com/cbti

Fulda, S., & Schulz, H. (2001). Cognitive dysfunction in sleep disorders. *Sleep Medicine Reviews, 5*(6), 423–445. https://doi.org/10.1053/smrv.2001.0157

Geng, C. (2021, September 29). *Menopause and insomnia: Link, duration, and remedies*. Www.medicalnewstoday.com. https://www.medicalnewstoday.com/articles/menopause-and-insomnia

Ghibellini, R., & Meier, B. (2022). The hypnagogic state: A brief update. *Journal of Sleep Research*. https://doi.org/10.1111/jsr.13719

Good Reads. (n.d.-a). *A quote by Mahatma Gandhi*. Www.goodreads.com. Retrieved November 3, 2023, from https://www.goodreads.com/quotes/1233102-each-night-when-i-go-to-sleep-i-die-and

Good Reads. (n.d.-b). *A quote by Ralph Waldo Emerson*. Www.goodreads.com. Retrieved November 3, 2023, from https://www.goodreads.com/quotes/711583-finish-each-day-before-you-begin-the-next-and-interpose

Hirshkowitz, M., Whiton, K., Albert, S. M., Alessi, C., Bruni, O., DonCarlos, L., Hazen, N., Herman, J., Adams Hillard, P. J., Katz, E. S., Kheirandish-Gozal, L., Neubauer, D. N., O'Donnell, A. E., Ohayon, M., Peever, J., Rawding, R., Sachdeva, R. C., Setters, B., Vitiello, M. V., & Ware, J. C. (2015). National Sleep Foundation's updated sleep duration recommendations: final report. *Sleep Health, 1*(4), 233–243. https://doi.org/10.1016/j.sleh.2015.10.004

Hopkins Medicine. (n.d.). *Sleepless nights? Try stress relief techniques*. Www.hopkins-

medicine.org. https://www.hopkinsmedicine.org/health/wellness-and-preven
tion/sleepless-nights-try-stress-relief-techniques

Kline, C. E. (2014). The bidirectional relationship between exercise and sleep. *American Journal of Lifestyle Medicine*, *8*(6), 375–379. https://doi.org/10.1177/1559827614544437

Kovacevic, A., Mavros, Y., Heisz, J. J., & Fiatarone Singh, M. A. (2018). The effect of resistance exercise on sleep: A systematic review of randomized controlled trials. *Sleep Medicine Reviews*, *39*, 52–68. https://doi.org/10.1016/j.smrv.2017.07.002

Lamberg, L. (2016). Treat chronic insomnia with CBT-I, says American College of Physicians. *Psychiatric News*, *51*(13), 1–1. https://doi.org/10.1176/appi.pn.2016.6b19

Lazarus, M., Shen, H.-Y. ., Cherasse, Y., Qu, W.-M. ., Huang, Z.-L. ., Bass, C. E., Winsky-Sommerer, R., Semba, K., Fredholm, B. B., Boison, D., Hayaishi, O., Urade, Y., & Chen, J.-F. . (2011). Arousal effect of caffeine depends on adenosine A2A receptors in the shell of the nucleus accumbens. *Journal of Neuroscience*, *31*(27), 10067–10075. https://doi.org/10.1523/jneurosci.6730-10.2011

Lee, S., Matsumori, K., Nishimura, K., Nishimura, Y., Ikeda, Y., Eto, T., & Higuchi, S. (2018). Melatonin suppression and sleepiness in children exposed to blue-enriched white LED lighting at night. *Physiological Reports*, *6*(24), e13942. https://doi.org/10.14814/phy2.13942

Li, H., Liu, Y., Xing, L., Yang, X., Xu, J., Ren, Q., Su, K.-P., Lu, Y., & Wang, F. (2020). Association of cigarette smoking with sleep disturbance and neurotransmitters in cerebrospinal fluid. *Nature and Science of Sleep*, *Volume 12*, 801–808. https://doi.org/10.2147/nss.s272883

Mariani, L. (2021, February 21). *"Your Future Depends On Your Dreams, So Go To Sleep" - Mesut Barazany - Be Your Best Self - A Daily Practice To Silence Your Inner Critic*. The People Alchemist. https://www.thepeoplealchemist.com/unlock-your-mind-transform-your-life/go-to-sleep/

Markwald, R. R., Iftikhar, I., & Youngstedt, S. D. (2018). Behavioral strategies, including exercise, for addressing insomnia. *ACSM's Health & Fitness Journal*, *22*(2), 23–29. https://doi.org/10.1249/FIT.0000000000000375

McMullin, M. F. (2012). Diagnosis and management of congenital and idiopathic erythrocytosis. *Therapeutic Advances in Hematology*, *3*(6), 391–398. https://doi.org/10.1177/2040620712458947

Mindful. (2020, September 30). *The ultimate guide to mindfulness for sleep*. Mindful. https://www.mindful.org/the-ultimate-guide-to-mindfulness-for-sleep/

Moore, P. (2021, April 30). Good sleep means more than getting enough hours. A consistent schedule matters, too. *Washington Post*. https://www.washington

post.com/lifestyle/wellness/enough-sleep-mental-health-circadian/2021/04/29/b9a2a396-a91e-11eb-bca5-048b2759a489_story.html

Morin, C. M., Bjorvatn, B., Chung, F., Holzinger, B., Partinen, M., Penzel, T., Ivers, H., Wing, Y. K., Chan, N. Y., Merikanto, I., Mota-Rolim, S., Macêdo, T., De Gennaro, L., Léger, D., Dauvilliers, Y., Plazzi, G., Nadorff, M. R., Bolstad, C. J., Sieminski, M., & Benedict, C. (2021). Insomnia, anxiety, and depression during the COVID-19 pandemic: an international collaborative study. *Sleep Medicine*, *87*, 38–45. https://doi.org/10.1016/j.sleep.2021.07.035

Naitoh, P., Kelly, T. L., & Englund, C. (1990). Health effects of sleep deprivation. *Occupational Medicine (Philadelphia, Pa.)*, *5*(2), 209–237. https://pubmed.ncbi.nlm.nih.gov/2203156/

National Heart, Lung, and Blood Institute. (2022, March 24). *How sleep works - Why is sleep important?* Www.nhlbi.nih.gov. https://www.nhlbi.nih.gov/health/sleep/why-sleep-important

National Institute on Aging. (2017). *A good night's sleep*. National Institute on Aging. https://www.nia.nih.gov/health/good-nights-sleep

Neckelmann, D., Mykletun, A., & Dahl, A. A. (2007). Chronic Insomnia as a Risk Factor for Developing Anxiety and Depression. *Sleep*, *30*(7), 873–880. https://www.ncbi.nlm.nih.gov/pmc/articles/PMC1978360/

NIH. (2022, March 24). *How sleep works - How much sleep is enough? | NHLBI, NIH*. Www.nhlbi.nih.gov. https://www.nhlbi.nih.gov/health/sleep/how-much-sleep

O'Connor, A. (2023, January 10). It's not just what you eat, but the time of day you eat it. *Washington Post*. https://www.washingtonpost.com/wellness/2023/01/10/meal-timing-big-meals/

O'Reilly, K. (2019, March 7). *Philips global sleep survey shows we want better sleep, but only if it comes easily*. Philips. https://www.philips.com/a-w/about/news/archive/standard/news/press/2019/20190307-philips-global-sleep-survey-shows-we-want-better-sleep-but-only-if-it-comes-easily.html

Park, S.-Y., Oh, M.-K., Lee, B.-S., Kim, H.-G., Lee, W.-J., Lee, J.-H., Lim, J.-T., & Kim, J.-Y. (2015). The effects of alcohol on quality of sleep. *Korean Journal of Family Medicine*, *36*(6), 294. https://doi.org/10.4082/kjfm.2015.36.6.294

Patel, A. K., & Araujo, J. F. (2018). *Physiology, sleep stages*. Nih.gov; StatPearls Publishing. https://www.ncbi.nlm.nih.gov/books/NBK526132/

Peng, J., Yuan, Y., Zhao, Y., & Ren, H. (2022). Effects of exercise on patients with obstructive sleep apnea: A systematic review and meta-analysis. *International Journal of Environmental Research and Public Health*, *19*(17), 10845. https://doi.org/10.3390/ijerph191710845

Pietilä, J., Helander, E., Korhonen, I., Myllymäki, T., Kujala, U. M., & Lindholm, H. (2018). Acute effect of alcohol intake on cardiovascular autonomic regulation during the first hours of sleep in a large real-world sample of Finnish employees: Observational Study. *JMIR Mental Health*, *5*(1), e23. https://doi.org/10.2196/mental.9519

Potter, G. D. M., Skene, D. J., Arendt, J., Cade, J. E., Grant, P. J., & Hardie, L. J. (2016). Circadian Rhythm and Sleep Disruption: Causes, Metabolic Consequences, and Countermeasures. *Endocrine Reviews*, *37*(6), 584–608. https://doi.org/10.1210/er.2016-1083

Quote Fancy. (n.d.). *Leo Tolstoy Quote: "Just as one candle lights another and can light thousands of other candles, so one heart illuminates another heart and c..."* Quotefancy.com. Retrieved November 7, 2023, from https://quotefancy.com/quote/851472/Leo-Tolstoy-Just-as-one-candle-lights-another-and-can-light-thousands-of-other-candles-so

Rossman, J. (2019). Cognitive-Behavioral Therapy for Insomnia: An Effective and Underutilized Treatment for Insomnia. *American Journal of Lifestyle Medicine*, *13*(6), 544–547. https://doi.org/10.1177/1559827619867677

Roth, T. (2007). Insomnia: definition, prevalence, etiology, and consequences. *Journal of Clinical Sleep Medicine : JCSM : Official Publication of the American Academy of Sleep Medicine*, *3*(5), S7-10. https://www.ncbi.nlm.nih.gov/pmc/articles/PMC1978319/

Rusch, H. L., Rosario, M., Levison, L. M., Olivera, A., Livingston, W. S., Wu, T., & Gill, J. M. (2018). The effect of mindfulness meditation on sleep quality: a systematic review and meta-analysis of randomized controlled trials. *Annals of the New York Academy of Sciences*, *1445*(1), 5–16. https://doi.org/10.1111/nyas.13996

Sagone, A. L. (1975). Smoking as a cause of erythrocytosis. *Annals of Internal Medicine*, *82*(4), 512. https://doi.org/10.7326/0003-4819-82-4-512

Sehgal, A., & Mignot, E. (2011). Genetics of sleep and sleep disorders. *Cell*, *146*(2), 194–207. https://doi.org/10.1016/j.cell.2011.07.004

Seol, J., Lee, J., Nagata, K., Fujii, Y., Joho, K., Tateoka, K., Inoue, T., Liu, J., & Okura, T. (2021). Combined effect of daily physical activity and social relationships on sleep disorder among older adults: cross-sectional and longitudinal study based on data from the Kasama study. *BMC Geriatrics*, *21*(1). https://doi.org/10.1186/s12877-021-02589-w

Staner, L. (2003). Sleep and anxiety disorders. *Dialogues in Clinical Neuroscience*, *5*(3), 249–258. https://www.ncbi.nlm.nih.gov/pmc/articles/PMC3181635/

Stutz, J., Eiholzer, R., & Spengler, C. M. (2018). Effects of evening exercise on sleep in healthy participants: A systematic review and meta-analysis. *Sports Medicine*, *49*(2), 269–287. https://doi.org/10.1007/s40279-018-1015-0

Suni, E. (2022). *What causes insomnia?* Sleepfoundation.org. https://www.sleepfoundation.org/insomnia/what-causes-insomnia

TalkPlus. (n.d.). *CBT for Insomnia*. https://www.talkplus.org.uk/downloads_folder/CBT_i.pdf

Taylor, D. J., Lichstein, K. L., & Durrence, H. H. (2003). Insomnia as a health risk factor. *Behavioral Sleep Medicine*, *1*(4), 227–247. https://doi.org/10.1207/s15402010bsm0104_5

Tosini, G., Ferguson, I., & Tsubota, K. (2016). Effects of blue light on the circadian system and eye physiology. *Molecular Vision*, *22*, 61–72. https://www.ncbi.nlm.nih.gov/pmc/articles/PMC4734149/

Troxel, W. M., Germain, A., & Buysse, D. J. (2012). Clinical management of insomnia with brief behavioral treatment (BBTI). *Behavioral Sleep Medicine*, *10*(4), 266–279. https://doi.org/10.1080/15402002.2011.607200

Troy, D. (2020, August). *Healthy sleep habits*. Sleep Education. https://sleepeducation.org/healthy-sleep/healthy-sleep-habits/

Turek, F., & Gillette, M. (2004). Melatonin, sleep, and circadian rhythms: rationale for development of specific melatonin agonists. *Sleep Medicine*, *5*(6), 523–532. https://doi.org/10.1016/j.sleep.2004.07.009

Versace, S., Pellitteri, G., Sperotto, R., Tartaglia, S., Da Porto, A., Catena, C., Gigli, G. L., Cavarape, A., & Valente, M. (2023). A state-of-art review of the vicious circle of sleep disorders, diabetes and neurodegeneration involving metabolism and microbiota alterations. *International Journal of Molecular Sciences*, *24*(13), 10615. https://doi.org/10.3390/ijms241310615

Veteran Training. (n.d.). *Insomnia action plan*. Retrieved November 7, 2023, from https://www.veterantraining.va.gov/apps/insomnia/resources/learn/documents/action_plan.pdf

Zhang, X., Li, W., & Wang, J. (2022). Effects of exercise intervention on students' test anxiety: A systematic review with a meta-analysis. *International Journal of Environmental Research and Public Health*, *19*(11), 6709. https://doi.org/10.3390/ijerph19116709

Made in United States
Orlando, FL
25 June 2024

48285189R00095